Atkins

The Ultimate Guide

©Kevin Case

Forward

First, I would like to thank you for purchasing "Atkins: The Ultimate Guide" and congratulate you for taking the leap to enhance your wellbeing and overall health.

The internet has been buzzing with the Atkins Diet, and rightly so. Its nutritional philosophy is pretty simple: eat fresh, natural and real food that fully nourishes your body and makes you feel good. This low carb diet reboots your system to get rid of all the negative eating habits such as sugar addiction and gives you another shot at finding balance in your life.

We are going to start by looking at why you need to start on the Atkins Diet by delving deeper into its philosophy and all the benefits you stand to gain by eating food just as nature intended.

Next, we are going to look at clean, fresh, healthy recipes bursting with flavour that are 100 present natural and that will rev up your metabolism.

To say that the Atkins Diet is life-changing would be an understatement. Following the Atkins Diet will allow you take control of your health and the benefits that will spill over to all parts of your life. Of course you can expect to see physical changes like definite weight loss, an increase in stamina and strength, and just generally feeling more comfortable in your own skin.

The Atkins Diet expounds on a practical and sustainable way to nourish our bodies to maintain lifelong health, physical performance and overall wellness, the same way our ancient ancestors thrived.

As you embark on this health journey, I hope it leads you to a life of pure health bliss and vitality as it has for so many other Atkins Diet devotees.

Table of Contents

Snack Recipes..581

The Truth About Weight Gain

"Our bodies are our gardens – our wills are our gardeners."

~William Shakespeare

Weight gain and obesity have become causes of health concerns in the western world. Obesity in particular is one of the leading causes of preventable death in the world today. Studies have been conducted to establish the reasons why the world population seems to be gaining weight. Research has shown, for instance, that the general weight of the population today, is much higher than it was in the 1960s.

What are the factors that have contributed to this turn of events and what are the intervention measures that can be instituted to control it? Studies have shown that although our children still engage in physical exercises, just like the children of yester years, they still add weight and in some cases get obese. For the older people, lack of exercise, among other issues has been cited a reason for weight gain or becoming fat.

Obesity and weight gain have been attributed to the foods we eat. Research shows that we have increased our food intake which unfortunately contains a higher percentage of sugar than what the world population used to ingest about fifty years ago. Also, the amount of fat that we eat has considerably increased. This coupled with lack of exercise have been cited as the leading causes of weight gain. It's an established fact that when we get large portions of fatty foods, creamy desserts, alcohol and soft drinks full of sugar, our calorie intake gets higher. With a higher calorie intake, we are expected to do a lot of exercises to burn the excess calories. If this is not done, there is a calorie pile up that leads to weight gain.

The solution to these problems lies in the ability to change our eating habits. One way of controlling unnecessary weight gain is the eating low carb foods. This way, the amount of calories in the food is closely controlled and helps in making one healthier.

Low Carb diets have been defined differently depending on whether the point of discussion is centered on the amount of calories derived from carbohydrates or the percentage of carbohydrates in a diet. Generally though, low carb diets can be described as those diets that help the body to derive between 5% to 45 % of calories from Carbohydrates. The normal percentage of calories that is supposed to be derived from Carbohydrates, according to the U.S. guidelines on health is between 50% to 65%. Therefore, a low carb diet refers to a conscious effort to try and limit the intake of foods with high carbohydrate levels, especially those that cause a significant rise in blood sugar.

Although the debate on the advantages of a low carb diet is still going on, it's true that the tolerance of carbohydrates in the body varies from person to person. This type of diet, then, will suit or benefit those who are sensitive or whose tolerance to carbohydrates is low. The approach is to encourage the reduction of the intake of carbohydrates to levels that the body can tolerate. This approach targets the reduction or elimination from our diets foods like potatoes, white rice, white flour and sugar from the diet.

The reduction of carbohydrates intake has been known to cause weight loss in people. To control this, a low carb diet should be closely monitored so that immediately signs of weight loss are noticed; the intake of carbohydrates is slowly increased until the body can control blood glucose. It's also advisable to embrace the Atkins Diet where the body generates energy from body fats instead of glucose. This leads the body into what is called fat adaptation. This adaptation encourages body metabolism which leads to improvement of stamina.

Energy from fat is long lasting unlike energy from glucose which quickly diminishes.

What is the Atkins Diet

Dr. Atkins, a well-known cardiologist, limited his patients' intake of sugar and carbohydrates. As a result, all of his patients successfully lost weight and kept it off – even though they had previously been unsuccessful on regular low-calorie diets!

The main premise of The Atkins Diet is restricting empty calorie carbohydrates in a systematic way, over the four phases that are outlined below.

The Atkins diet consists of a four-phase eating plan. The foods you eat vary depending on what phase you are in and your own personal **metabolism**. The four phases of the Atkins diet include:

Phase 1-Induction - This is the first phase of the Atkins diet, and should be implemented for **a minimum of 2 weeks**. It is also considered the most restrictive phase. In other words, phase one allows you to eat very little to no carbohydrates. You are limited to only **20 grams** per day. The carbs you are allowed to eat consist of salad and other non-starchy vegetables. This is where the most dramatic weight loss occurs.

Phase 2-Ongoing Weight Loss - Phase two allows you to add some carbohydrates to your diet. In this phase, carbs are increased to 25 grams per day. Each week, you can increase the number of carbs you eat by **five** grams. So, the second week of phase two, you can have 30 grams of carbs. The third week you can consume 35 grams of carbs and so on. You continue on the course of slowly increasing carbohydrates until your body stops losing weight. When that occurs, you subtract five grams of carbohydrates from your daily intake. This level will allow you to maintain your weight. Here you can add back certain vegetables, berries, nuts, and seeds, slightly increasing carb intake without stopping weight loss. This is the longest stage of the diet, and you stay here until you are about 10 pounds from your weight loss goal.

Phase 3-Pre-Maintenance - In this phase, you transition from weight loss to weight maintenance. You can increase your carbohydrate allowance by 10-gram increments each week as long as you continue to keep the weight off. If weight loss stops, you cut carbs again, just enough to maintain a steady weight loss until you reach your goal.

Phase 4-Lifetime Maintenance - The final phase allows you to select from a wide variety of foods, while still limiting the amount of carbohydrates you eat. It is this phase that allows you to continue to keep your weight down as well as allows you to eat more foods than in the previous phases. In this lifetime maintenance stage your target carb intake is 45 to 100 grams per day.

The Benefits of The Atkins Diet

When you choose a diet, you want to make sure there are plenty of positive benefits beyond losing weight. You want to be healthier overall by eating in the manner the diet instructs you to eat on a daily basis. You also want to be able to follow the plan for life instead of just a few weeks or months. The benefits of the Atkins diet will provide the healthy daily plan you can implement for life.

You may not realize that eating carbs can increase the chance of negative health issues. By reducing the volume of carbs daily that you eat, some medical conditions you often experience may occur less often. The frequency of headaches, joint pain, and trouble concentrating will diminish when you reduce the intake of carbs. This may help you reduce the amount of pain medicine you take when the pain of headaches and joints go away. So you will feel healthier and save money on medicine by the benefits of a low carb diet.

Often when you diet mood swings can cause the process to be difficult. The highs and lows of mood and energy can cause you to binge eat. Another benefit of the Atkins diet is the balancing of mood and energy. Actually the body gets more consistent energy from protein and other nutrients than from carbs. Carbs bring on short term energy spurts that will drop your energy level quickly once the carbs are digested. By lowering the volume of carbs you eat, your energy will come from other nutrients that are more consistent energy reducing mood and energy swings.

If you enjoy exercise and want to tone and build muscle tissue which helps fight fat in your body, a low carb diet can help. After a workout your muscles are very sensitive to insulin and do not need as many carbs as some people may think. By eating a low carb diet, your muscles after a workout will draw in more amino acids from your meal. The amino acids will help the muscles heal from the workout quicker and burn more fat.

The impact or prevention of diabetes can be helped by a low carb diet. If you have diabetes a low carb diet may help balance your insulin level more throughout the day. If you have family members with diabetes and want to avoid getting the disease yourself, a low carb diet is a good healthy way to naturally balance your insulin.

So as you can see, there are many benefits of the Atkins diet beyond just losing weight. You will see an improvement in your weight but you will also have more energy and feel healthier. That is the goal of losing weight as well; to be healthier.

Eating more vegetables and proteins as well as fruits and nuts can be a good start to the Atkins Diet, provided you are in the second and consecutive phases. Completely cut out your intake of breads, sweets, and items made from white flour and white sugar. In the following chapter you will find a full meal plan as well as hundreds of delicious recipes.

Enjoy!

1 FULL Month Meal Plan

You've heard it said; 'failure to plan is planning to fail.' Whether you are only cooking for one or for your entire family, taking the time to sit and plan for what you are going to eat for the coming week will not just save you time, money and effort; it will also enhance your healthy eating habits.

Four reasons why you should have a meal plan:

- You will culture healthy eating habits

The main premise of The Atkins Diet is to eat foods that are going to burn more calories than you consume, as well as boost your immune system and protect you from chronic disease. When you have a carefully set out meal plan, you won't need to resort to ordering takeout as you will have healthy food waiting for you at home.

Habit is second to nature and as you get used to planning healthy meals, you will soon forget about the processed and inflammatory foods that used to slow you down.

- You become an informed shopper

The specific ingredients listed in the recipes you are going to make will teach you the healthiest ingredients that you need to buy. Forget about overly processed food that has got no nutritional value, you focus will now shift to fresh, natural, nutrient dense foods.

- You will save time and money

When you know exactly what you are going to cook, you will shop for ingredients more efficiently and thus save more money. You won't also have to waste time brainstorming on what to cook as it's already planned.

- You will eat a variety of food

Planning your meals will allow you to eat something new almost every day, if not every day, instead of eating one thing all week. If you have a family, they are sure to love this method and it will give them something to look forward to every day.

Meal Plan – Week One			
	Monday	Tuesday	Wednesday
Breakfast	Vanilla Chia Oatmeal	Bacon Avocado Breakfast Muffins	Easy Pancakes
Lunch	Coco Shrimps and Chili Dip	BLT Roll	Hearty Portobello Burgers
Dinner	Duck Breast with Balsamic Vinegar	Oriental Shrimp Soup	Zucchini Soup with Crunchy Cured Ham
Thursday	**Friday**	**Saturday**	**Sunday**
Mozzarella, Red Pepper & Bacon Frittata	Cream Cheese Pancakes	Mug Bread	Anaheim pepper Gruyere Waffles
Salmon Salad in Avocado Cups	Mediterranean Pecorino Romano Breaded Cutlets	Baked Pork Chops in Sweet-Sour Marinade	Zucchini and Mascarpone Rolls
Curried Coconut Chicken Fingers	Smoky Pork Cassoulet	Creamy Tarragon Chicken	Chicken Stir-Fry

Meal Plan – Week Two			
	Monday	**Tuesday**	**Wednesday**
Breakfast	Lime Peppermint Smoothie	Eggs with Motley Peppers and Zucchini	Kale, Peppers and Crumbled Feta Omelet (Slow Cooker)
Lunch	Chicken and Cucumber Salad	Zesty Herbed Chicken	Turkey Meatballs
Dinner	Slow Cooker Thai Fish Curry	Seared Ribeye Steak	Beanless Chili con Carne
Thursday	**Friday**	**Saturday**	**Sunday**
Fisherman's Breakfast	Nonpareil Bacon Waffles	Mini Ham Omelets Muffins	Guacamole Bacon and Eggs Breakfast
Salmon Burgers	Curry-Spiced Salad	Cauliflower and Cheese Chowder	Beef Sausage, Bacon & Broccoli Casserole
Burger Patties	Easy Roast Tomato Sauce	Baked Buttered Chicken	Macadamia Crusted Lamb Chops

Meal Plan - Week Three			
	Monday	**Tuesday**	**Wednesday**
Breakfast	Cashew Chocolate & Orange Smoothie	Autumn Pumpkin Bread	Bacon Avocado Breakfast Muffins
Lunch	Pizza in Mushroom Cups	Sausage and Cheese Bombs	Chicken Cordon Bleu
Dinner	Ratatouille	The Perfect Baked Chicken Wings	Cheeseburger Soup Indulgence
Thursday	**Friday**	**Saturday**	**Sunday**
Pork and Sage Breakfast Burgers	Sour and Spicy Goat Skewers	Ham and Cheese Omelet	Baked Parmesan-Almond Zucchini
Spring Roll in a Bowl	Green Salad	Spicy Chicken Thighs	Chicken Alfredo Pizza
Ground Chicken Satay	Turkey Leg Roast	Baked Herb Salmon Fillets	Chicken and Mushroom Stew

Meal Plan – Week Four			
	Monday	**Tuesday**	**Wednesday**
Breakfast	Baked Broccoli with Mushrooms and Parmesan	Flax-Almond Coated Cheddar	Fast Protein and Peanut-Butter Pancakes
Lunch	Roquefort Spinach, Zoodles and Bacon Salad	Cheesy Pizza	Pordenone Cauliflower Lasagna
Dinner	Cheeseburger Casserole	Curried Madras Lamb	Slow Cooker Oxtail Stew
Thursday	**Friday**	**Saturday**	**Sunday**
Hemp Muffins with Walnuts	Millet Gingerbread Mash	Baked Ham and Kale Scrambled Eggs	Egg Pesto Scramble
BBQ Chicken Soup	Baked Creamy Cauliflower-Broccoli Chicken	Slow Cooker Roast and Chicken Stew	Bolognese Squash Spaghetti
Bacon Layered Lasagna	Atkins-Friendly Pad Thai	Pork and Shrimp Stuffed Peppers	Sirloin Tip Cut with Cilantro Sauce

Breakfast Recipes

Breakfast Berry Mug Cake

Ingredients

2 organic eggs

¼ cup vanilla syrup, sugar-free

2 tbsp. melted ghee

2 tbsp. organic cream cheese, set at room temperature

¼ tsp. almond flour

¼ cup raspberries and strawberries, chopped

For the whipped cream topping:

¼ cup whipped cream

½ tbsp. vanilla syrup, sugar-free

Directions

1. Place the eggs, vanilla syrup, melted ghee, and cream cheese into a blender and blend until all the ingredients are well-mixed.

2. Transfer the batter into an oven-safe mug and then mix the flour and berries into the batter. Stir well.

3. Place in the oven and cook for 4 minutes on high.

4. While waiting for the cake to cook, place the whipping cream and vanilla syrup in a blender and blend until the cream stiffens.

5. Serve the mug cake with a generous scoop of the vanilla of whipped cream on top.

Serves 1

Nutritional Information

Calories 463

Net Carbs 40.4g

Fats 25.0g

Protein 13.2g

Coco Cereal

Ingredients

3 tsp. organic butter

½ cup coconut shreds, unsweetened

¾ cup toasted walnuts, roughly chopped

¾ cup toasted macadamia nuts, roughly chopped

2 cups almond milk

1/8 tsp. salt

½ tbsp. stevia (optional)

Directions

1. Melt the butter in a pot over medium fire. Add the toasted nuts to the pot and stir for 2 minutes.

2. Add the shredded coconuts into the pot and continue stirring to make sure to not burn the ingredients.

3. Drizzle with stevia (if using) and then pour the milk into the pot. Stir again and turn the heat off.

4. Allow to rest for 10 minutes to allow the ingredients to soak in the milk before consuming.

Makes 2-3

Nutritional Information

Calories 515

Net Carbs 14.4g

Fats 50.3g

Protein 6.5g

Fiber 7.3g

Sweet n' Creamy Egg Bowl

Ingredients

2 organic eggs

1/3 cup heavy cream, preferably organic

½ tbsp. stevia

2 tbsp. organic butter

1/8 tsp. cinnamon, ground

Directions

1. In a small bowl, whisk the eggs, whipping cream, and sweetener.

2. Melt the organic butter in a pan over medium heat and then pour in the egg mixture.

3. Stir and cook until the eggs starts to thicken and then transfer into a bowl.

4. Sprinkle with cinnamon on top before serving.

Serves 1

Nutritional Information

Calories 561

Net Carbs 6.4g

Fats 53.6g

Protein 15g

Fiber 0g

Pump-Cakes

Ingredients

¼ hazelnuts flour

2 tbsp. egg white protein

1 tsp. baking powder

1 tbsp. chai masala mix

½ cup pumpkin puree

3 free-range eggs

1 cup coconut cream

1 tbsp. stevia

Organic butter for cooking

Coconut cream for topping

Directions

1. In a bowl, combine the hazelnut flour, egg white protein, baking protein, and chai masala mix, and Servia. Stir well and set aside.

2. Using another mixing bowl, combine the pumpkin puree, eggs, and coconut cream. Blend the ingredients together until frothy using a hand mixer.

3. Take the dry ingredients and then gradually whisk into the bowl with the pumpkin mixture.

4. The batter should be quite thick, but pourable. If the batter is too thick, add a few tablespoons of water.

5. Melt the butter in a non-stick pan over low heat.

6. Ladle the batter on the hot. Cover and allow to cook for about 3 minutes on each side.

7. Serve the pump-cakes warm with a spoon of coconut cream on top.

Serves 2-3

Nutritional Information

Calories 626

Net Carbs 17.1g

Fats 58.3g

Protein 16g

Fiber 7.2g

Protein Loaded Bread

Ingredients

12 eggs whites, preferably organic

1 cup whey protein

4 oz. softened cream cheese

Directions

1. Set the oven at 325F.

2. Pour the egg white and whey protein into a bowl and whisk using a hand mixer until the whites are stiff.

3. Gently fold in the cream cheese into the mixture and pour over 2 greased bread pans.

4. Place in the oven to cook for 40 minutes or until the bread is golden brown.

5. Allow the bread to cook before cutting into slices. Serve or store the bread in the freezer.

Makes 2 loaves (18 slices)

Nutritional Information

per 2 slices

Calories 144

Net Carbs 0.9g

Fats 11.5g

Protein 9.4g

Fiber 0g

Protein French Bread

Ingredients

8 slices protein loaded bread

2 organic eggs

¼ cup coconut milk

1 tsp. vanilla extract

1 tsp. cinnamon powder

coconut oil for frying

For the syrup:

½ cup organic butter

½ cup sugar replacement

½ cup almond milk, unsweetened

Directions

1. Prepare the syrup by heating the butter on a saucepan. Wait for the butter to boil (careful not to burn) and then pour the sugar replacement and almond milk into the sauce pan. Whisk the ingredients together until smooth. Set aside to cool before transferring into a storage container.

2. In a bowl, whisk together the eggs coconut milk, extract, and cinnamon.

3. Dip the bread slices into the mixture and place on a hot non-stick skillet with coconut oil

4. Toast until the breads are brown on each side.

5. Do the same procedure until you've toasted all the bread slices.

6. Serve the French toasts with a drizzle of the prepared syrup on top.

Serves 4

Nutritional Information

Calories 265

Net Carbs 1.5g

Fats 24.5g

Protein 11.0g

Fiber 0g

Anchovy, Spinach and Asparagus Omelet

Ingredients

2 organic eggs

3/4 cup of spinach

2 oz. anchovy in olive oil

4 marinated asparagus

Celtic Sea salt

Freshly ground black pepper

Directions

1. Preheat the oven to 375 F.
2. In the bottom of the baking pan place the anchovy.
3. In a bowl, beat the eggs and pour on top of the fish. Add the spinach and the chopped asparagus on top.
4. Season with salt and pepper to taste.
5. Bake in preheated oven for about 10 minutes.
6. Serve hot.

Servings: 2

Cooking Times

Total Time: 15 minutes

Amount Per Serving

Calories 83,

41

Fat 4,91g

Carbs 2,28g

Fiber 0,86g

Sugar 0,23g

Protein 7,7g

Autumn Pumpkin Bread

Ingredients

3 egg whites

1/2 cup coconut milk

1 1/2 cup almond flour

1/2 cup pumpkin puree

2 tsp. baking powder

1 1/2 tsp. Pumpkin pie spice

1/2 tsp. Kosher Salt

coconut oil for greasing

Directions

1. Preheat your oven to 350F. Grease a standard bread loaf pan with melted coconut oil.

2. Sift all dry ingredients into a large bowl.

3. In another bowl, add pumpkin puree and coconut milk and mix well. In a separate bowl, beat the egg whites. Fold in egg whites and gently fold into the dough.

4. Spread the dough into the prepared bread pan.

5. Bake the bread for 75 minutes. Once ready, remove bread from the oven and let cool.

6. Slice and serve.

Servings: 8

Cooking Times

Total Time: 1 hour and 25 minutes

Amount Per Serving

Calories 197

Fat 16,69g

Carbs 8,19g

Fiber 3,31g

Sugar 1,89g

Protein 7,24g

Batter Coated Cheddar Cheese

Ingredients

1 large egg

2 slice Cheddar cheese (3.55 oz.)

1 tsp. ground walnuts

1 tsp. ground flaxseed

2 tsp. almond flour

1 tsp. hemp seeds

1 Tbsp. olive oil

Salt and pepper to taste

Directions

1. In a small bowl, whisk an egg together with the salt and pepper.

2. Heat a tablespoon of olive oil in a frying pan, on medium heat.

3. In a separate bowl, mix the ground flaxseed with the ground walnuts, hemp seeds and the almond flour.

4. Coat the cheddar slices with the egg mix, then roll in the dry mix and fry cheese for about 3 minutes on each side. Serve hot.

Servings: 1

Cooking Times

Total Time: 13 minutes

Amount Per Serving

Calories 509,

Fat 46,19g

Carbs 2,65g

Fiber 0,79g

Protein 21,98g

Chicken Sausage and Pepper Jack Pie

Ingredients

5 egg yolks

1 1/2 chicken sausage

3/4 cup Pepper Jack cheese

1/4 cup coconut flour

2 tsp. lime Juice

1/2 tsp. dried basil

1/4 tsp. baking soda

4 Tbsp. coconut oil

2 Tbsp. coconut water

Kosher salt to taste

Directions

1. Preheat oven to 350F.
2. In a frying pan add the sausages and cook on medium high heat 3-4 minutes. Set aside.
3. Measure out the dry ingredients into a bowl.
4. Separate 5 egg yolks from the whites, then discard of the whites.
5. Beat the egg yolks about 4-5 minutes. Add in coconut oil, coconut water, and lime juice. Continue to beat again until smooth and creamy.
6. Mix the wet ingredients into the dry ingredients slowly. At last, add cheese into the batter.
7. Measure out the batter into 2 ramekins. Poke the sausages into the batter.
8. Bake in preheated oven for 25 minutes. Once ready, serve hot.

Servings: 5

Cooking Times: 40 minutes

Amount Per Serving

Calories 294

Fat 24,78g

Carbs 7,66g

Fiber 0,34g

Protein 11g

Cashew Chocolate & Orange Smoothie

Ingredients

1 cup cashew milk

1 handful of arugula leaves

1 Tbsp. chocolate whey protein powder

1/8 tsp. orange extract

Ice cubes

Directions

1. Place all ingredients in your blender and blend until well united and smooth. Add extra ice and serve.

Servings: 1

Cooking Time: 5 minutes

Amount Per Serving

Calories 44

Fat 1,05g

Carbs 7,1g

Fiber 2,49g

Sugar 4,4g

Protein 3,97g

Coffee Atkins-chino

Ingredients

1 cup cold coffee

1/3 cup heavy cream

1/4 tsp. xanthan gum

1 tsp. pure vanilla extract

2 Tbsp. Xylitol

6 ice cubes

Directions

1. Place all ingredients in your blender. Blend until all unite well and become smooth. Serve.

Servings: 1

Cooking Times: 5 minutes

Amount Per Serving

Calories 287

Fat 29,37g

Carbs 2,74g

Fiber 0g

Protein 1,91g

Cheesy Boiled Eggs

Ingredients

3 eggs

2 Tbsp. almond butter, no-stir

2 Tbsp. softened cream cheese

1 tsp. whipping cream

Salt and pepper to taste

Directions

1. In a small saucepan hard boil the eggs.
2. When ready, wash the eggs with cold water, peel and chop them. Place eggs in a bowl; add in the butter, cream cheese and whipping cream.
3. Mix well and add salt and pepper to taste. Serve.

Servings: 2

Cooking Time: 20 minutes

Amount Per Serving

Calories 212

Total Fat 19,88g

Total Carbohydrates 0,75g

Protein 7,74g

Mahón Kale Sausage Omelet Pie

Ingredients

10 eggs

1 1/2 cup Mahón cheese (or Cheddar)

3 chicken sausages

3 cups raw chopped Kale leaves

2 1/2 cup mushrooms, chopped

1 Tbsp. garlic powder

2 tsp. hot sauce

1/2 tsp. black pepper and celery seed

salt and pepper to taste

Directions

1. Preheat oven to 400F.
2. Chop up your sausage and mushroom thin and place them in a cast iron skillet. Cook on a medium-high heat for 2-3 minutes.
3. While the sausages are cooking, chop your spinach up. Add in a skillet the mushrooms and spinach.
4. In a meanwhile, in a bowl mix eggs with black pepper and celery seed, hot sauce, and spices. Scramble them well.
5. Mix your sausages, spinach, and mushrooms so that the spinach can wilt fully. Add salt and pepper to taste.
6. Finally, add the cheese to the top.
7. Pour your eggs over the mixture and mix everything well.
8. Stir the mixture for a few seconds, and then put your cast iron skillet in the oven. Bake for 10-12 minutes, and then broil the top for 3-4 minutes.
9. Let cool for a while, cut into 8 slices and serve hot.

Servings: 8

Cooking Times: 25 minutes

Amount Per Serving

Calories 266

Total Fat 17,76g

Total Carbohydrates 7,67g

Fiber 0,92g

Protein 19,37g

Monterey Bacon-Scallions Omelet

Ingredients

2 eggs

2 slices cooked bacon

1/4 cup scallions, chopped

1/4 cup Monterey jack cheese

salt and pepper to taste

1 tsp. lard

Directions

1. In a frying pan heat lard in on medium-low heat. Add the eggs, scallions and salt and pepper to taste.

2. Cook for 1-2 minutes; add the bacon and sauté 30 - 45 seconds longer. Turn the heat off on the stove.

3. On top of the bacon place a cheese. Then, take two edges of the omelet and fold them onto the cheese. Hold the edges there for a moment as the cheese has to partially melt. Make the same with the other egg and let cook in a warm pan for a while.

4. Serve hot.

Servings: 2

Cooking Times

Total Time: 15 minutes

Amount Per Serving

54

Calories 321

Fat 28,31g

Carbs 1,62g

Fiber 0,33g

Protein 14,37g

Smoked Turkey Bacon and Avocado Muffins

Ingredients

5 eggs

6 slices smoked turkey bacon

1/2 cup almond flour

2 medium Avocados

1/2 cup Cheddar cheese

1 1/2 cup coconut milk

3 spring onions

1 tsp. minced garlic

2 tsp. dried parsley

1/4 tsp. red chili powder

1 1/2 Tbsp. lemon juice

1/4 cup flaxseed

1 1/2 Tbsp. Metamucil powder

1 tsp. baking powder

2 Tbsp. butter

salt and pepper to taste

Directions

1. Preheat oven to 350F.
2. In a frying pan over medium-low heat, cook the bacon with the butter until crisp. Add the spring onions, cheese, and baking powder.
3. In a bowl, mix together coconut milk, eggs, Metamucil powder, almond flour, flax, spices and lemon juice. Switch off the heat and let cool. Then, crumble the bacon and add all of the fat to the egg mixture.
4. Clean and chop avocado and fold into the mixture.

5. Measure out batter into a cupcake tray that's been sprayed or greased with nonstick spray and bake for 25-26 minutes.

6. Once ready, let cool and serve hot or cold.

Servings: 16
Cooking Times: 40 minutes

Amount Per Serving

Calories 184
Fat 16,4g
Carbs 5,51g
Fiber 2,7g
 Protein 5,89g

Sour Cream Cheese Pancakes

Ingredients

2 eggs

1/4 cup cream cheese

1 Tbsp. coconut flour

1 tsp. ground ginger

1/2 cup liquid Stevia

coconut oil

sugar-free maple syrup

Directions

1. In a deep bowl, beat together all of the ingredients until smooth.

2. Heat up a frying skillet with oil on medium-high. Ladle the batter and pour in hot oil.

3. Cook on one side and then flip. Top with a sugar-free maple syrup and serve.

Servings: 2

Cooking Times

Total Time: 15 minutes

Amount Per Serving

Calories 170

Total Fat 13,71g

Carbs 4,39g

Fiber 0,14g

Protein 6,9g

Spicy Cauliflower with Sujuk Sausages

Ingredients

4 cups frozen cauliflower

8 oz. sujuk sausages sliced (or red pastrami)

1 green pepper, chopped

1 tsp. Cajun seasoning

1/2 onion, chopped

2 Tbsp. minced garlic

2 Tbsp. olive oil

Directions

1. In a frying pan, sauté onion with olive oil for 2-3 minutes.

2. Squeeze the liquid from chopped cauliflower and add it to the pan. Sauté the cauliflower with onion 5-10 minutes.

3. Add in Cajun seasoning and mix. Add in chopped sujuk sausages or pastrami and green peppers.

4. Toss and cook until about 5 minutes. Transfer to the plates. Serve.

Servings: 4

Cooking Times

Total Time: 20 minutes

Amount Per Serving

Calories 181

Fat 10,21g

Carbs 9,52g

Fiber 2,77g

Protein 14g

Strawberry Marjoram Smoothie

Ingredients

1/4 cup fresh or frozen strawberries

2 fresh marjoram leaves

2 Tbsp. heavy cream

1 cup unsweetened coconut milk

1 Tbsp. sugar-free vanilla syrup

1/2 tsp. pure vanilla extract

ice cubes (optional)

Directions

1. Place all ingredients in your blender and mix until become smooth.
2. If you wish you can add the ice cubes. Serve.

Servings: 1

Cooking Time: 5 minutes

Amount Per Serving

Calories 292, 35

Fat 29,75g

Carbs 6,78g

Protein 2,84g

Vesuvius Scrambled Eggs with Provolone

Ingredients

2 large eggs

3/4 cup Provolone cheese

1.76 oz. air-dried salami

1 tsp. fresh rosemary (chopped)

1 Tbsp. Olive oil

Salt and pepper to taste

Directions

1. In a small pan with olive oil fry the chopped salami.
2. In the meantime, in a small bowl whisk the eggs, then add the salt, pepper and fresh rosemary.
3. Add in the provolone cheese and mix well with a fork.
4. Pour the egg mixture to the pan with salami and cook for about 5 minutes. Serve hot.

Servings: 2

Cooking Time: 10 minutes

Amount Per Serving

Calories 374

Total Fat 30,32g

Total Carbs 2,43g

Fiber 0,27g

Protein 22,45g

Pizza Waffles

Ingredients

Parmesan cheese (4 tablespoons)

Psyllium husk powder (1 tablespoon)

Baking powder (1 teaspoon)

Salt

Cheddar cheese (3 oz.)

Eggs (4, large)

Almond flour (3 tablespoons)

Butter (1 tablespoon, organic)

Italian seasoning (1 teaspoon)-you may use a teaspoon of your preferred spices

Tomato sauce (1/2 cup)

Directions

1. Add all ingredients to a bowl except cheese and tomato sauce. Use mixer or immersion blender to combine until mixture is thick.

2. Heat waffle iron and use mixture to make two waffles.

3. Place waffles onto a lined baking sheet and top with tomato sauce and cheese (divide evenly). Broil for 3 minutes or until cheese melts.

4. Serve.

Servings: 2

Nutritional Information

Calories 525

Net Carbs 5g

Fats 41.5g

Protein 29g

Fiber 5.5g

Pancakes and Syrup

Ingredients

For pancakes:

Eggs (4, large)

Erythritol (2 tablespoons)

Baking soda (1/2 teaspoon)

Nut butter of your choice (3/4 cup)

Coconut milk (1/3 cup)

Ghee (2 tablespoons)

Cinnamon powder (1 teaspoon)

For Syrup:

Maple extract (2 tablespoons, sugar-free)

Sukrin Fiber Syrup (1/2 cup)

Directions

1. Add ingredients for syrup to a jar and use spoon to stir until combined thoroughly. Cover jar and put aside until needed.

2. Put eggs, erythritol, baking soda, nut butter, coconut milk and cinnamon powder in a food processor and pulse until blended.

3. Heat ghee in a non-stick skillet and add batter to pot, use about ¼ cup per pancake. Cook until pancake sets then flip and finish cooking; place on a plate.

4. Repeat with remaining batter and plate.

5. Top with syrup and serve.

Servings: 5

Nutritional Information

Calories 401

Net Carbs 3.6g

Fats 32.5g

Protein 12.8g

Fiber 5.3g

Cheesy Bacon and Chive Omelet

Ingredients

Bacon fat (1 teaspoon)

Cheddar cheese (1 oz.)

Salt

Bacon (2 slices, cooked)

Eggs (2, large)

Black pepper

Chives (2 stalks)

Directions

1. Beat eggs together and add pepper and salt to taste. Chop chives and shred cheese.

2. Heat skillet and cook bacon fat until hot.

3. Add eggs to pot and top with chives. Cook until edges start to set then add bacon and cook for 30-60 seconds.

4. Add cheese and use spatula to fold in half. Press to seal and flip over.

5. Warm and serve immediately.

Servings: 1

Nutritional Information

Calories 463

Net Carbs 1g

Fats 39g

Protein 24g

Fiber 0g

Breakfast Quiche

Ingredients

Coconut oil (3 tablespoons)

5 whole eggs

8 slices of bacon, cooked and chopped

100ml cream

Baby spinach, roughly chopped (2 cups)

Red pepper, chopped (1 cup)

Green pepper, chopped (1 cup)

Yellow onion, chopped (1 cup)

2 cloves of garlic, minced

Mushrooms, chopped (1 cup)

100g cheddar cheese, grated

salt to taste

Directions

1. Preheat oven at 375F

2. In a large bowl, mix all vegetables including the mushrooms together.

3. In another small bowl, whisk the 5 eggs with the cream

4. Carefully scoop the veggie mixture into a muffin pan coated with cooking spray, top with egg and cheese filling up to ¾ of the muffin tins. Sprinkle with chopped bacon on top.

5. Place in the oven to bake for 15 minutes or until the top of the quiche are firm.

6. Let it cook for a few minutes before serving.

Servings: 5

Nutritional Information

Calories: 210

Net Carbs: 5g

Fat: 13g

Protein: 6g

Bacon Avocado Breakfast Muffins

Ingredients

Bacon (5 slices)

Almond flour (1/2 cup)

Psyllium husk powder (1 ½ tablespoons)

Colby Jack cheese (4.5 oz.)

Garlic (1 teaspoon, diced)

Chives (1 teaspoon, dried)

Salt

Lemon juice (1 ½ tablespoons)

Eggs (5)

Butter (2 tablespoons, organic)

Flaxseed meal (1/4 cup)

Avocados (2, cubed)

Spring onions (3)

Cilantro (1 teaspoon, dried)

Red chili flakes (1/4 teaspoon)

Coconut milk (1 ½ cup, from box)

Black Pepper

Baking powder (1 teaspoon)

Directions

1. Add flour, spices, lemon juice, eggs, flaxseed meal and coconut milk to a bowl. Mix together until thoroughly combined.
2. Heat a skillet and cook bacon until crispy then add the butter and avocado.
3. Add mixture to batter in bowl and mix together.
4. Set oven to 350 F and grease cupcake molds.

5. Add batter to molds and bake for 26 minutes. Take from oven and cool before removing from mold.
6. Serve. Store leftovers in fridge.

Servings: 16

Nutritional Information

Calories 163
Net Carbs 1.5g
Fats 14.1g
Protein 6.1g
Fiber 3.3g

Chicharrones con Huevos (Pork Rind & Eggs)

Ingredients

Bacon (4 slices)

Pork Rinds (1.5 oz.)

Avocado (1, cubed)

Onion (1/4, chopped)

Salt

Eggs (5)

Tomato (1, chopped)

Jalapeno pepper (2, seeds removed and chopped)

Cilantro (1/4 cup, chopped)

Black pepper

Directions

1. Heat skillet and cook bacon until slightly crisp. Remove from pot and put aside on paper towels.

2. Add pork rinds to pot along with onion, tomatoes, pepper and cook for 3 minutes until onions are soft and clear.

3. Add cilantro, stir together gently and add eggs. Scramble eggs and then add avocado and fold.

4. Serve.

Servings: 3

Nutritional Information

Calories 508

Net Carbs 5g

Fats 43g

Protein 24.7g

Fiber 5.3g

Red Pepper, Mozzarella and Bacon Frittata

Ingredients

Olive oil (1 tablespoon)

Parsley (2 tablespoons, chopped)

Mozzarella cheese (4 oz., cubed)

Bell pepper (1, red, chopped)

Heavy cream (1/4 cup)

Salt

Bacon (7 slices)

Bella mushrooms (4 caps, large)

Basil (1/2 cup, chopped)

Goat cheese (2 oz., grated)

Eggs (9)

Parmesan cheese (1/4 cup, grated)

Black pepper

Directions

1. Set oven to 350 °F.

2. Chop red pepper, bacon, basil and mushroom. Slice mozzarella into cubes and put aside.

3. Heat olive oil in a skillet until it slightly smokes then add bacon and cook for 5 minutes until browned.

4. Add red pepper and cook for 2 minutes until soft. While pepper cooks, add cream, parmesan cheese, eggs and black pepper to a bowl and whisk to combine.

5. Add mushrooms to pot, stir and cook for 5 minutes until soaked in fat. Add basil, cook for 1 minute then add mozzarella.

6. Put in egg mixture and use spoon to move ingredients around so that the egg gets on the bottom of pan.

7. Top with goat cheese and place in oven for 8 minutes then broil for 6 minutes.

8. Use knife to pry frittata edges from pan and place on a plate and slice.

9. Serve.

Servings: 6

Nutritional Information

Calories 408

Net Carbs 2.4g

Fats 31.2g

Protein 19.2g

Fiber 0.8g

Cheese and Sausage Pies

Ingredients

Cheddar cheese (3/4 cup, grated)

Coconut oil (1/4 cup)

Egg yolks (5)

Rosemary (1/2 teaspoon)

Baking soda (1/4 teaspoon)

Chicken sausage (1 ½)

Coconut flour (1/4 cup)

Coconut milk (2 tablespoons)

Lemon juice (2 teaspoons)

Cayenne pepper (1/4 teaspoon)

Kosher salt (1/8 teaspoon)

Directions

1. Set oven to 350 F.

2. Chop sausage, heat skillet and cook sausage. While sausages cook combine all dry ingredients in a bowl. In another bowl combine lemon juice, oil and coconut milk. Add liquids to dry mixture and add ½ cup of cheese; fold to combine and put into 2 ramekins.

3. Add cooked sausages to batter and use spoon to push into mixture.

4. Bake for 25 minutes until golden on top. Top with leftover cheese and broil for 4 minutes.

5. Serve warm.

Servings: 2

Nutritional Information

Calories 711

Net Carbs 5.8g

Fats 65.3g

Protein 34.3g

Fiber 11.5g

Vanilla Chia Oatmeal

Ingredients

Chia seeds (1/4 cup)

Coconut flakes (1/3 cup, unsweetened)

Vanilla (1 teaspoon, sugar free)

Almond milk (1 cup, unsweetened)

Stevia extract (10 drops)

Coconut (1/4 cup, shredded, unsweetened)

Almonds (1/3 cup, flaked)

Heavy whipping cream (1/2 cup)

Erythritol (2 tablespoons)

Directions

1. Place almond and coconut flakes in a pot and toast for 3 minutes until fragrant.
2. Place toasted ingredients into a bowl along with chia seeds, erythritol and shredded coconut; mix together to combine.
3. Top with milk and stir. You can use hot or cold milk based on your preference.
4. Add vanilla and stevia, stir and set aside for 5-10 minutes.
5. Serve. May be topped with fresh berries.

Servings: 2

Nutritional Information

Calories 359

Net Carbs 5g

Fats 30.4g

Protein 9.4 g

Fiber 10.5g

Breakfast Berry Shake

Ingredients

Mixed berries (3/4 cup)

Almond milk (1 cup)

All-natural peanut butter (1 tablespoon)

Protein powder (1 tablespoon)

Cinnamon powder (1/4 teaspoons)

Ginger, minced (1/4 teaspoons)

Directions

1.   Place all the ingredients in a blender and mix until smooth.

Servings: 3

Nutritional Information

Calories: 319

Net Carbs: 9g

Fat: 15g

Protein: 28g

Breakfast Tacos

Ingredients

Eggs (6)

Bacon (3 strips)

Cheddar cheese (1 oz., shredded)

Mozzarella cheese (1 cup, shredded)

Butter (2 tablespoons)

Avocado (1/2, cubed)

Salt

Black pepper

Directions

1. Cook bacon until crisp, put aside until needed.

2. Heat a non-stick pan and place 1/3 cup mozzarella into pan and cook for 3 minutes until browned around the edges. Place a wooden spoon across a bowl or pot and use tongs to lift cheese 'taco from pot. Repeat with leftover cheese.

3. Melt butter in a skillet and scramble eggs; use pepper and salt to season.

4. Spoon eggs into hardened shells and top with avocado and bacon.

5. Top with cheddar and serve.

Servings: 2

Nutritional Information

Calories 443

Net Carbs 3g

Fats 36.2g

Protein 25.7 g

Fiber 1.7g

Raspberry & Cacao Breakfast Pudding

Ingredients

Cacao powder (1 tablespoon)

Raspberry (1/4 cups)

Chia seeds (3 tablespoon)

Almond milk (1 cup)

Agave or Xylitol (1 teaspoon)

Directions

1. In a small bowl, combine the almond milk and cacao powder. Stir well.

2. Add the chia seeds to the bowl and let it rest for 5 minutes.

3. Using a fork, fluff the chia and cacao mixture and then place in the fridge to chill for at least 30 minutes.

4. Serve with raspberries and a drizzle of agave on top

Servings: 1

Nutritional Information

Calories 230

Net Carbs 4g

Fats 20g

Protein 15 g

Orange Cinnamon Scones

Ingredients

For Scones:

Heavy cream (1/3 cup)

Butter (1/4 cup, unsalted, cubed)

Coconut oil (2 tablespoons)

Golden Flaxseed (1 tablespoon)

Cinnamon (1 ½ teaspoons)

Xanthan (1/4 teaspoon)

Salt (1/4 teaspoon)

Coconut flour (8 tablespoons)

Erythitol (1/4 cup)

Eggs (2)

Maple syrup (2 tablespoons)-recipe above

Baking powder (1 ½ teaspoons)

Vanilla (1 teaspoon)

Stevia (1/4 teaspoon)

Orange zest (from 1 orange)

For Icing:

Stevia (20 drops)

Orange juice (1 tablespoon)

Coconut butter (1/4 cup)

Directions

1. Set oven to 400 °F.

2. Place all dry ingredients in a bowl except xanthan and 1 tablespoon flour. Add butter and oil to dry mix and stir to combine.

3. Combine sweetener and eggs until thoroughly mixed and light in color. Put in maple syrup, remaining flour, xanthan gum, heavy cream and vanilla; mix until combined and thick.

4. Add wet mixture to dry, reserving 2 tablespoons of liquids, mix together and add cinnamon and use hands to form mixture into dough. Shape into a ball and press into a cake like shape. Slice into 8 pieces.

5. Place onto a lined baking sheet and use reserved liquid to brush the top of scones.

6. Bake for 15 minutes, remove from oven and cool.

7. Prepare icing and drizzle over scones before serving.

Servings: 8

Nutritional Information

Calories 232

Net Carbs 3.3g

Fats 20g

Protein 3.3 g

Fiber 4.3g

Buttermilk Seed Rusks

Ingredients

½ cup butter, melted

1 cup buttermilk

4 eggs

1 cup almond flour

1 cup ground flax

2 cups desiccated coconut

1 cup mixed seeds

2 ½ tsp. baking powder

1 tsp. salt

½ cup Xylitol

Directions

1. Preheat oven at 350F

2. In a bowl, combine the yogurt, butter, and eggs.

3. Slowly add the dry ingredients and stir well to make a batter.

4. Carefully transfer the mixture into a baking tray and cook in the oven for 45 minutes.

5. Allow to cool down before slicing it into 30 rusk shapes.

6. Place on a wire rack upside down, and cook in the oven again for 90 minutes at 210F.

Servings: 30

Nutritional Info (1 rusk)

Calories: 119

Net Carbs: 17g

Fat: 3g

Protein: 2g

Caprese Stack

Ingredients

3 slices mozzarella cheese

2 large slices of tomato

4 fresh basil leaves

salt and pepper

1 tsp. olive oil

Directions

1. On a plate, stack the mozzarella cheese, tomato, and basil.

2. Season with salt and pepper and drizzle with olive oil

Nutritional Info (per stack)

Calories: 186

Net Carbs: 5g

Fat: 10g

Protein: 6g

Easy Pancakes

Ingredients

1 tbsp. melted butter

2 eggs

5 tbsp. full-fat milk

1 tbsp. xylitol

½ tsp. salt

2 tbsp. coconut flour

1 tbsp. almond flour

½ tsp. baking powder

Directions

1. In a bowl, whisk the eggs with the milk, salt, xylitol, and melted butter (room temp.)

2. Add the coconut and almond flour to the mixture, along with the baking powder. Mix well.

3. Heat a non-stick pan over medium fire and scoop 3 tbsp. of the batter to make pancakes.

4. Flip the pancake when bubbles start to form and cook until golden brown.

5. Serve with ½ cup of berries on the side.

Servings: 2

Nutritional Info (1 pc.)

Calories: 194

Net Carbs: 30g

Fat: 13g

Protein: 31g

Mug Bread

Ingredients

1 tbsp. coconut flour

3 tbsp. almond flour

1 tsp. baking powder

1 whole egg

1 tsp. melted butter

3 tbsp. water

a pinch of salt

Directions

1. Add all the dry ingredients in a bowl then add the egg and water and mix well make sure there are no lumps in your mixture.

2. Pour the melted butter in the cup you are going to use. You can also use the cup to melt the butter to begin with, but make sure not to over heat the butter; 5 seconds in the microwave should be more than enough. Now swirl the butter around the cup make sure to coat the inside of the cup then pour the butter into the bread mix and combine.

3. Pour the mix in your cup and microwave for 1.5 minutes. if you are planning on doubling the mix I would suggest using a bigger wider mug or the mix will not cook all the way through. Don't microwave for more than 3 min or the mix will end up hard.

4. Once you have removed it from the mug, you can then slice it into rounds and place it in the toaster to crisp it up a little.

Servings: 1

Nutritional Info (1 serving)

Calories: 238

Net Carbs: 2.6g

Fat: 19g

Protein: 13g

Veggie Scramble

Ingredients

4 egg whites

1 egg yolk

2 tbsp. almond milk

1 cup spinach

1 tomato, chopped

½ white onion, chopped

3 fresh basil leaves, chopped

salt and pepper to taste

ghee

Directions

1. In a bowl, whisk the egg yolk and whites with the milk. Stir well.

2. Heat the ghee on a pan over medium heat. Add the onions and sauté until fragrant.

3. Throw in the tomato to the pan with the spinach and cook until the spinach is almost wilted.

4. Pour the egg mixture to the spinach and cook until firm or until the egg sets. Stir constantly.

5. Season with salt and pepper.

6. Serve warm

Nutritional Info (per serving)

Calories: 203

Net Carbs: 18g

Fat: 5g

Protein: 20g

Egg Pesto Scramble

Ingredients

3 eggs

1 tbsp. pesto sauce

1 tbsp. olive oil

2 tbsp. sour cream

Directions

1. Whisk the eggs in a bowl and season with salt and pepper.

2. Heat a non-stick pan over low heat. Drizzle with olive oil and pour the eggs. Constantly whisk the eggs while cooking.

3. Add the pesto mixture to the eggs and stir well.

4. Turn off the fire and mix in the sour cream. Combine well.

5. Serve with 1/2 cup mashed avocado.

Servings: 1

Nutritional Info (per serving)

Calories: 467

Net Carbs: 3.3g

Fat: 41.5g

Protein: 20.4g

Cheesy Low Carb Bread

Ingredients

125g full-fat cream cheese

1 cup cheddar cheese, grated

3 large eggs

1 tsp. apple cider vinegar

2 cups almond flour

2 tsp. baking powder

1 tsp. mustard powder

1 tsp. salt

Directions

1. Preheat oven at 375F

2. Combine all the ingredients in a bowl with a hand mixer, except the cheddar cheese.

3. Add the cheddar cheese to the mixture and combine using a spatula or a fork. Be careful not to mush the cheese.

4. Line a bread tin with well-greased baking paper and bake in the oven for 45 minutes.

Nutritional Info (per serving)

Calories: 495

Net Carbs: 6.5g

Fat: 9.6g

Protein: 19.7g

Lemon Cheesecake Breakfast Mousse

Ingredients

3 tbsp. cream cheese

1 tbsp. lemon juice

50ml heavy cream (look for those with zero carbs)

100ml Yoghurt

1tbsp. Xylitol

1/8 tsp. salt

2 tbsp. whey protein

Directions

1. Blend cream cheese and lemon juice in a bowl until smooth.

2. Add heavy cream and blend until whipped. Gently add in yoghurt.

3. Taste and adjust sweetener if needed.

4. Serve with ¼ cup berry coulis.

Berry Breakfast Shake

Ingredients

¾ cup mixed berries

1 cup almond milk

1 tbsp. all-natural peanut butter

1 tbsp. protein powder

¼ tsp. cinnamon powder

¼ tsp. ginger, minced

Directions

1. Place all the ingredients in a blender and mix until smooth.

Servings: 1

Nutritional Info (per serving)

Calories: 319

Net Carbs: 9g

Fat: 15g

Protein: 28g

Cacao and Raspberry Pudding

Ingredients

1 tbsp. cacao powder

¼ cup raspberry

3 tbsp. chia seeds

1 cup almond milk

1 tsp. agave

Directions

2. In a small bowl, combine the almond milk and cacao powder. Stir well.

3. Add the chia seeds to the bowl and let it rest for 5 minutes.

4. Using a fork, fluff the chia and cacao mixture and then place in the fridge to chill for at least 30 minutes.

5. Serve with raspberries and a drizzle of agave on top

Coco and Blueberry Smoothie

Ingredients

½ cup blueberries

½ cup coconut cream

1 tbsp. coconut oil

½ cup almond milk, vanilla flavor

3 ice cubes

Directions

1. Place all the ingredients in a blender and mix until you achieve a smooth consistency.

Servings: 2

Nutrition info for one serving:

Calories 295

Fat 24g

Protein 13g

Carbs 6g

Fibre 1g

Creamy Chocolate Milk

Ingredients

16 ounces unsweetened almond milk

1 teaspoon xylitol

4 ounces heavy cream

1 scoop Whey Chocolate Isolate powder

1/2 cup crushed ice (optional: add if you like a thick drink, but the flavour will be less intense.)

Directions

1.   Put all ingredients in blender and blend until smooth.

Servings: 2

Nutrition info for one serving:

Calories 292

Fat 25g

Protein 15g

Carbs 5g

Blueberry Almond Smoothie

Ingredients

16 ounces unsweetened almond milk

1 teaspoon xylitol

4 ounces heavy cream

1/4 cup frozen unsweetened blueberries

1 scoop Whey Vanilla protein powder

Directions

1. Put all ingredients in blender and blend until smooth.

2. Add a little water if it becomes too thick.

3. Measure those blueberries as they add more carbs.

Servings: 2

Nutrition info for one serving:

Calories 302

Fat 25g

Protein 15g

Carbs 6g

Fibre 1g

Mozzarella, Red Pepper & Bacon Frittata

Ingredients

Olive oil (1 tablespoon)

Parsley (2 tablespoons, chopped)

Mozzarella cheese (4 oz., cubed)

Bell pepper (1, red, chopped)

Heavy cream (1/4 cup)

Salt

Bacon (7 slices)

Bella mushrooms (4 caps, large)

Basil (1/2 cup, chopped)

Goat cheese (2 oz., grated)

Eggs (9)

Parmesan cheese (1/4 cup, grated)

Black pepper

Directions

1. Set oven to 350 F.
2. Chop red pepper, bacon, basil and mushroom. Slice mozzarella into cubes and put aside.
3. Heat olive oil in a skillet until it slightly smokes then add bacon and cook for 5 minutes until browned.
4. Add red pepper and cook for 2 minutes until soft. While pepper cooks, add cream, parmesan cheese, eggs and black pepper to a bowl and whisk to combine.
5. Add mushrooms to pot, stir and cook for 5 minutes until soaked in fat. Add basil, cook for 1 minute then add mozzarella.
6. Put in egg mixture and use spoon to move ingredients around so that the egg gets on the bottom of pan.

7. Top with goat cheese and place in oven for 8 minutes then broil for 6 minutes.

8. Use knife to pry frittata edges from pan and place on a plate and slice.

9. Serve.

Servings: 6

Nutritional Information

Calories 408
Net Carbs 2.4g
Fats 31.2g
Protein 19.2g
Fiber 0.8g

Rosemary, Sausage & Cheese Pies

Ingredients

Cheddar cheese (3/4 cup, grated)

Coconut oil (1/4 cup)

Egg yolks (5)

Rosemary (1/2 teaspoon)

Baking soda (1/4 teaspoon)

Chicken sausage (1 ½)

Coconut flour (1/4 cup)

Coconut milk (2 tablespoons)

Lemon juice (2 teaspoons)

Cayenne pepper (1/4 teaspoon)

Kosher salt (1/8 teaspoon)

Directions

1. Set oven to 350 F.

2. Chop sausage, heat skillet and cook sausage. While sausages cook combine all dry ingredients in a bowl. In another bowl combine lemon juice, oil and coconut milk. Add liquids to dry mixture and add ½ cup of cheese; fold to combine and put into 2 ramekins.

3. Add cooked sausages to batter and use spoon to push into mixture.

4. Bake for 25 minutes until golden on top. Top with leftover cheese and broil for 4 minutes.

5. Serve warm.

Servings: 2

Nutritional Information

Calories 711

Net Carbs 5.8g

Fats 65.3g

Protein 34.3g

Fiber 11.5g

Kale Sausage Omelet Pie

Ingredients

10 eggs

1 1/2 cup Mahón cheese (or Cheddar)

3 chicken sausages

3 cups raw chopped Kale leaves

2 1/2 cup mushrooms, chopped

1 Tbsp. garlic powder

2 tsp. hot sauce

1/2 tsp. black pepper and celery seed

Salt and pepper to taste

Directions

1. Preheat oven to 400F.
2. Chop up your sausage and mushroom thin and place them in a cast iron skillet. Cook on a medium-high heat for 2-3 minutes.
3. While the sausages are cooking, chop your spinach up. Add in a skillet the mushrooms and spinach.
4. In a meanwhile, in a bowl mix eggs with black pepper and celery seed, hot sauce, and spices. Scramble them well.
5. Mix your sausages, spinach, and mushrooms so that the spinach can wilt fully. Add salt and pepper to taste.
6. Finally, add the cheese to the top.
7. Pour your eggs over the mixture and mix everything well.
8. Stir the mixture for a few seconds, and then put your cast iron skillet in the oven. Bake for 10-12 minutes, and then broil the top for 3-4 minutes.
9. Let cool for a while, cut into 8 slices and serve hot.

Servings: 8

Cooking Time: 25 minutes

Amount Per Serving

Calories 266

Fat 17,76g

Carbs 7,67g

Fiber 0,92g

Protein 19,37g

Bacon, Scallions & Monterey Omelet

Ingredients

2 eggs

2 slices cooked bacon

1/4 cup scallions, chopped

1/4 cup Monterey jack cheese

salt and pepper to taste

1 tsp. lard

Directions

1. In a frying pan heat lard in on medium-low heat. Add the eggs, scallions and salt and pepper to taste.

2. Cook for 1-2 minutes; add the bacon and sauté 30 - 45 seconds longer. Turn the heat off on the stove.

3. On top of the bacon place a cheese. Then, take two edges of the omelet and fold them onto the cheese. Hold the edges there for a moment as the cheese has to partially melt. Make the same with the other egg and let cook in a warm pan for a while.

4. Serve hot.

Servings: 2

Cooking Time: 15 minutes

Amount Per Serving

Calories 321

Fat 28,31g

Carbs 1,62g

Fiber 0,33g

Sugar 0,55g

Protein 14,37g

Bacon, Avocado & Smoked Turkey Muffins

Ingredients

5 eggs

6 slices smoked turkey bacon

1/2 cup almond flour

2 medium Avocados

1/2 cup Cheddar cheese

1 1/2 cup coconut milk

3 spring onions

1 tsp. minced garlic

2 tsp. dried parsley

1/4 tsp. red chili powder

1 1/2 Tbsp. lemon juice

1/4 cup flaxseed

1 1/2 Tbsp. Metamucil powder

1 tsp. baking powder

2 Tbsp. butter

salt and pepper to taste

Directions

1. Preheat oven to 350F.

2. In a frying pan over medium-low heat, cook the bacon with the butter until crisp. Add the spring onions, cheese, and baking powder.

3. In a bowl, mix together coconut milk, eggs, Metamucil powder, almond flour, flax, spices and lemon juice. Switch off

the heat and let cool. Then, crumble the bacon and add all of the fat to the egg mixture.

4. Clean and chop avocado and fold into the mixture.

5. Measure out batter into a cupcake tray that's been sprayed or greased with nonstick spray and bake for 25-26 minutes.

6. Once ready, let cool and serve hot or cold.

Servings: 16

Cooking Time: 40 minutes

Amount Per Serving

Calories 184

Fat 16,4g

Carbs 5,51g

Fiber 2,7g

Sugar 0,54g

Protein 5,89g

Cream Cheese Pancakes

Ingredients

2 eggs

1/4 cup cream cheese

1 Tbsp. coconut flour

1 tsp. ground ginger

1/2 cup liquid Stevia

coconut oil

sugar-free maple syrup

Directions

1. In a deep bowl, beat together all of the ingredients until smooth.

2. Heat up a frying skillet with oil on medium-high. Ladle the batter and pour in hot oil.

3. Cook on one side and then flip. Top with a sugar-free maple syrup and serve.

Servings: 16

Cooking Time: 15 minutes

Amount Per Serving

Calories 170, 78

Fat 13,71g

Carbs 4,39g

Fiber 0,14g

116

Protein 6,9g

Pumpkin Flaxseed Muffins

Ingredients

1 egg

1 1/4 cup flaxseeds (ground)

1 cup pumpkin puree

1 Tbs pumpkin pie spice

2 Tbs coconut oil

1/2 cup sweetener of your choice

1 tsp baking powder

2 tsp cinnamon

1/2 tsp apple cider vinegar

1/2 tsp vanilla extract

salt to taste

Directions

1. Preheat your oven to 360°F.
2. First, grind the flaxseeds for several seconds.
3. Put together all the dry ingredients and stir.
4. Then, add your pumpkin puree and mix to combine.
5. Add the vanilla extract and the pumpkin spice.
6. Add in coconut oil, egg and apple vinegar. Add sweetener of your choice and stir again.
7. Add a heaping tablespoon of batter to each lined muffin or cupcake and top with some pumpkin seeds.
8. Bake for about 18 - 20 minutes. Serve hot.

Servings: 10

Cooking Times: 20 minutes

Nutrition Facts (per serving)

Carbs: 3g

Fiber: 1g

Protein: 1g

Fat: 5.34g

Calories: 43

Baked Ham and Kale Scrambled Eggs

Ingredients

5 ounces ham diced

2 medium eggs

1 green onion, finely chopped

1/2 cups kale leaves, chopped

1 garlic clove, crushed

1 green chilli, finely chopped

4 ready-roasted peppers

pinch cayenne pepper

1 Tbsp olive oil

1/2 can water

Directions

1. Heat oven to 360F.

2. Heat the oil in a small ovenproof frying pan. Add green onion and cook for 4-5 mins until softened.

3. Stir in the garlic and chilli, and cook for a couple mins more.

4. Add the 1/2 cup water. Season well and stir through the ready-roasted peppers and ham. Bring to a simmer and cook for 10 mins.

5. Add the kale, stirring through to wilt.

6. In a small bowl, beat the eggs with a pinch of cayenne and pour in frying pan together with other ingredients.

7. Transfer the frying pan to the oven and bake for 10 mins.

8. Serve hot.

Servings: 2

Cooking Times

Preparation Time: 10 minutes

Cooking Time: 30 minutes

Total Time: 2 hours and 20 minutes

Nutrition Facts (per serving)

Carbs: 3,8g

Fiber: 0,8g

Protein: 22g

Fat: 15,74g

Calories: 251

Bell Pepper and Ham Omelet

Ingredients

4 large eggs

1 cup green pepper (chopped)

1/4 lb ham, cooked and diced

1 green onion, diced

1 tsp coconut oil

salt and freshly ground pepper to taste

Directions

1. Wash and chop vegetables. Set aside.

2. Into a small bowl beat the eggs. Set aside.

3. Heat non-stick skillet over medium heat and add coconut oil. Pour half of the beaten eggs into the skillet.

4. When the egg has partially set, add half of the vegetables and ham to one half of the omelet and continue to cook until the egg is almost fully set.

5. Fold the empty half over top of the ham and veggies using a spatula.

6. Cook for 2 minutes more and then serve.

7. Serve hot.

Servings: 2

Nutrition Facts (per serving)

Carbs: 6,8g

Protein: 21,88g

Fat: 12g

Calories: 225,76

Chia Flour Pancakes

Ingredients

1 cup Chia flour

2 tsp sweetener of your choice

1 egg, beaten

1 Tbsp coconut butter or oil

1/2 cup coconut milk (canned)

Directions

1. In a medium bowl, combine the flour and sugar. Add the egg, milk and coconut butter. Mix well until make a smooth batter.

2. Grease a non-stick skillet and heat over medium-high heat. Drop a heaping tablespoon of batter onto the hot surface.

3. When bubbles form on the surface of the scones, use a spatula to turn them and then cook about 2 minutes per side.

4. Serve hot.

Servings: 6

Cooking Time: 15 minutes

Nutrition Facts (per serving)

Carbs: 4,65g

Protein: 2,46g

Fat: 3,5g

Calories: 59

Choco Moko Chia Porridge

Ingredients

3 Tbs Chia Seeds

1 cup almond milk, unsweetened

2 tsp cocoa powder

1/4 cup raspberries -fresh or frozen

2 Tbsp almond, ground

Sweetener of your choice (optional)

Directions

1. Mix and stir the almond milk and the cocoa powder together.
2. Add the Chia Seeds in the mixture.
3. Mix well with a fork.
4. Place the mixture in a fridge for 30 minutes.
5. Serve with raspberries and ground almonds on the top. (optional)

Servings: 2

Inactive Time: 30 minutes. Cooking Time: 5 minutes

Nutrition Facts (per serving)

Carbs: 15,2g

Fiber: 11,28g

Protein: 5,47g

Fat: 9,62g

Calories: 150,1

Coffee Flaxseed Dream Breakfast

Ingredients

3 Tbsp flaxseed, ground

1/2 cup strong black coffee, unsweetened

2 1/2 Tbsp coconut flakes, unsweetened

1 Tbsp coconut oil, melted

Sweetener of your choice to taste

1/2 cup water (optional)

Directions

1. In a bowl, combine the flaxseed and the coconut flakes.
2. Add the melted coconut oil, then pour the hot coffee over it and mix.
3. If it is too thick, add a little water.
4. At the end, add the sweetener of your choice to taste.
5. Ready! Enjoy!!

Servings: 1

Nutrition Facts (per serving)

Carbs: 1,52

Fiber: 0,9g

Protein: 1,48g

Fat: 22,1

Calories: 246,43

Crimini Mushroom with Boiled Eggs Breakfast

Ingredients

14 Crimini mushroom, finely chopped

8 large eggs, hard-boiled, chopped

6 slices bacon or pancetta

1 spring onion, diced

Salt and ground black pepper to taste

Directions

1. In a frying pan cook bacon. Reserve a bacon fat in the pan. Chop up bacon pieces and set aside.

2. In a deep saucepan, hard-boil the eggs. When ready, wah, clean, shell and chop into bite-size pieces.

3. In a frying pan cook the spring onion with remaining bacon fat over medium-high heat.

4. Add the Crimini mushrooms and sauté another 5-6 minutes.

5. Blend the eggs, bacon and cook together. Adjust salt and ground black pepper to taste.

6. Serve.

Servings: 6

Cooking Time: 20 minutes

Nutrition Facts (per serving)

Carbs: 2,43g

Fiber: 1,5g

Protein: 11,32

Fat: 13

Calories: 176

Anaheim pepper Gruyere Waffles

Ingredients

1 small Anaheim pepper

3 eggs

1/4 cup cream cheese

1/4 cup Gruyere cheese

1 Tbsp. coconut flour

1 tsp. Metamucil powder

1 tsp. baking powder

Salt and pepper to taste

Directions

1. In a blender, mix together all ingredients except for the cheese and Anaheim pepper.

2. Once the ingredients are mixed well, add cheese and pepper. Blend well until all ingredients are unit well.

3. Heat your waffle iron; pour on the waffle mix and cook 5-6 minutes.

4. Serve hot.

Servings: 2

Cooking Times

Total Time: 15 minutes

Amount Per Serving

131

Calories 223

Fat 17g

Carbs 5,53g

Fiber 0,33g

Sugar 1,56g

Protein 11,6g

Egg Whites and Spinach Omelet

Ingredients

5 egg whites

2 Tbsp almond milk

1 zucchini, shredded

1 cup spinach leaves, fresh

2 Tbs spring onion, chopped

2 cloves garlic

Olive oil

Basil leaves, fresh, chopped

Salt and ground black pepper to taste

Directions

1. Wash and chop the vegetables

2. In a bowl, beat the egg whites and the almond milk.

3. In a greased frying pan with olive oil, cook the vegetables (spinach, zucchini, spring onion) just for one to two minutes.

4. Put the vegetables on the side, grease the pan again with olive oil and pour the eggs. Cook until the eggs are firm. Add the vegetables on one side and cook for two minutes more. Adjust salt and pepper to taste.

5. Decorate with basil leaves and serve.

Servings: 2

Cooking Times

133

Total Time: 15 minutes

Nutrition Facts (per serving)

Carbs: 5,78g

Fiber: 1,58g

Protein: 11,08g

Fat: 1,56g

Calories: 70,8

Fast Protein and Peanut-Butter Pancakes

Ingredients

1 scoop of low-carb protein powder

2 eggs

2 Tbsp of natural peanut butter

2 Tbsp flaxseed

2 Tbsp water

olive oil for greasing

Directions

1. In a bowl, mix protein powder, eggs, peanut butter, water and flaxseeds.

2. Grease with olive oil and heat a large non-stick frying pan over medium heat.

3. Laddle a batter mixture and cook for 2 minutes per side or until bubbles appear on surface. Transfer to a plate.

4. Serve hot.

Servings: 1

Cooking Time: 15 minutes

Nutrition Facts (per serving)

Carbs: 13,78g

Fiber: 8,48g

Protein: 17,8g

Fat: 23,59g

135

Calories: 406,41

Guacamole Bacon and Eggs Breakfast

Ingredients

4 slices bacon or pancetta

2 Tbsp heavy cream

2 Tbsp avocado oil

4 eggs

salt and peppet to taste

Directions

1. In a bowl, beat eggs with heavy cream and salt and ground pepper to taste.
2. Pour egg mixture over bacon and cook for 2-3 minutes.
3. Flip bacon and eggs on other side and cook for 1 minute more.
4. Serve and enjoy!

Servings: 4

Cooking Time: 13 minutes

Nutrition Facts (per serving)

Carbs: 0,66g

Fiber: 0g

Protein: 9,28g

Fat: 22,43g

Calories: 292

Hemp Muffins with Walnuts

Ingredients

2 1/2 cup Hemp flour

1 1/2 cup walnuts, chopped

1/2 cup sweetener of your choice

4 Tbsp extra-virgin olive oil

1 tsp vanilla extract

2 tsp baking powder

1 tsp baking soda

Directions

1. Preheat oven to 345F.

2. In a small bowl whisk olive oil, sweetener of your choice and vanilla.

3. In a separate bowl, combine hemp flour, baking powder and baking soda. Add in chopped walnuts and toss to coat.

4. Add olive oil mixture to the flour mixture and stir slightly.

5. Spoon a batter into 12 muffin cups, filling 3/4 full.

6. Bake 18 - 20 minutes. Allow to cool 10 minutes in the muffin pan, then turn out onto a wire rack to cool completely. Serve.

Servings: 12

Cooking Time: 30 minutes

Nutrition Facts (per serving)

Carbs: 25,18g

138

Fiber: 4,43g

Protein: 7,75g

Fat: 16,45g

Calories: 270

Baked Pancetta and Eggs

Ingredients

6 slices Pancetta, crumbled

8 eggs

3/4 cup Cheddar cheese, grated

3/4 cup heavy cream

salt and pepper to taste

olive oil for greasing

Directions

1. Preheat the oven to 350 degrees F. Grease a big baking dish with olive oil.

2. In a bowl, beat the eggs with shredded Cheddar cheese and cream, and season with salt and pepper to taste.

3. Crumble Pancetta evenly over the egg mixture. Put the baking dish in a preheated oven.

4. Bake for 15 minutes.

5. Serve immediately.

Servings: 6

Cooking Times: 20 minutes

Nutrition Facts (per serving)

Carbs: 1,49g

Fiber: 0g

Protein: 12,5g

Fat: 22,03g

Calories: 254,89

Bilberry Coconut Mush

Ingredients

1/4 cup coconut flour

1 cup coconut milk

1/4 cup ground flaxseed

1 tsp vanilla extract

1 tsp cinnamon

Liquid sweetener of your choice

Toppings

1 cup bilberries

2 Tbs shaved coconut

2 Tbs pumpkin seeds

Directions

1. In a saucepan heat the coconut milk. Add in coconut flour, cinnamon and flaxseed and whisk.

2. Add in vanilla extract and liquid sweetener of your choice. Cook for 10 minutes stirring constantly. Remove from heat and let cook for 2-3 minutes.

3. Decorate with fresh bilberries, pumpkin seeds and shaved coconut to taste.

Servings: 2

Cooking Times

Total Time: 5 minutes

Nutrition Facts (per serving)

Carbs: 16,4g

Fiber: 1,69

Protein: 2,86g

Fat: 22,4f

Calories:445

Boiled Eggs with Mascarpone and Bacon

Ingredients

2 large eggs

2 Tbsp Mascarpone cheese

2 Tbs crumbled bacon

1 Tbs coconut butter

salt and pepper to taste

Directions

1. Hard boil the eggs; bring water to a boil over medium-high heat, then cover, remove from the heat and set aside for 10 minutes.

2. Wash, peel and chop boiled eggs and place them in a large bowl.

3. Add the butter and the Mascarpone cheese, mix well. Adjust salt and pepper to taste.

4. Serve.

Servings: 2

Cooking Time: 15 minutes

Nutrition Facts (per serving)

Carbs: 0,91g

Fiber: 0g

Protein: 11,1g

Fat: 22,84g

Calories: 328,34

Flax-Almond Coated Cheddar

Ingredients

4 oz Cheddar cheese, 2 slices

1 large egg

1 tsp almond flour or ground almonds

1 Tbsp flaxseed, ground

1 tsp hemp seeds

1 Tbsp Olive oil

Salt and pepper to taste

Directions

1. In a non-stick frying pan heat a tablespoon of olive oil.

2. In a bowl, combine the almond flour, the ground flaxseed and the hemp seeds.

3. In a separate bowl, beat an egg together with the salt and pepper.

4. Coat the cheddar slices first with the egg mix and then with the dry mix. Fry cheese for about 3 minutes on each side. Serve hot.

Servings: 2

Cooking Time: 15 minutes

Nutrition Facts (per serving)

Carbs: 4,28g

Fiber: 2,83g

Protein: 17,91g

Fat: 22,37g

Calories: 358,62

French Almond Toast

Ingredients

4 eggs

1/4 cup coconut milk

2 Tbsp coconut oil (melted)

6 slices almond bread

2 tsp sweetener of your choice (optional)

1/2 tsp cinnamon powder

1 tsp organic vanilla extract

salt and pepper (per taste)

Directions

1. Whisk coconut milk, sweetener of your choice, eggs, organic vanilla extract, salt and cinnamon.

2. Soak each slice of almond bread (or any gluten free vegan Hemp & Seed bread) in egg mixture.

3. In a frying pan, heat the coconut oil over high heat; cook each slice of bread three minutes or until golden. Transfer toast to the plate lined with paper.

4. Serve hot.

Servings: 6

Nutrition Facts (per serving)

Carbs: 11,13g

Fiber: 0,57g

148

Protein: 6,56g

Fat: 10,2g

Calories: 162,6

Pork and Sage Breakfast Burgers

Ingredients

1 lb ground pork

2 Tbsp fresh sage, chopped

1 tsp garlic powder

1 tsp cayenne pepper

salt and pepper to taste

2 Tbsp granular sweetener of your choice

olive oil for greasing

Directions

1. In a large bowl, combine all ingredients except olive oil. Use hands to mix thoroughly.

2. Form into 8 evenly burgers.

3. Grease with olive oil your large frying pan over medium heat.

4. Add burger and cook about 3 to 4 minutes per side.

5. Ready. Serve and enjoy!!

Servings: 4

Cooking Time: 15 minutes

Nutrition Facts (per serving)

Carbs: 0,78g

Fiber: 0,44g

Protein: 19,29g

Fat: 22,17g

Calories: 302,21

Quick & Easy Flax "Muffins"

Ingredients

4 Tbsp ground flax meal

1 egg

1 Tbs of heavy whipping cream

1 tsp organic vanilla extract

2 tsp sweetener of your choice

1 pinch salt

coconut butter

cocoa powder (optional)

Directions

1. Mix all ingredients in a microwave safe bowl; stir to combine well.

2. Place a bit of coconut butter on the top. Microwave for one and a half minutes.

3. If you want, you can add a splash of unsweetened cocoa powder.

4. Ready! Serve! Enjoy!

Servings: 1

Cooking Times

Total Time: 5 minutes

Nutrition Facts (per serving)

152

Carbs: 10,24g

Fiber: 1,36g

Protein: 8,21g

Fat: 8,4g

Calories: 160,51

Millet Gingerbread Mash

Ingredients

1 cup millet flour (or any kind of whole grain flour)

4 cups water

1/2 tsp ground ginger

1/4 tsp ground allspice

1/8 tsp ground nutmeg

1/4 tsp ground cardamom

1/4 tsp ground coriander

1 1/2 Tbs ground cinnamon

1 tsp ground cloves

sweetener of your choice (optional)

Directions

1. In a medium saucepan bring water to boiling and cook the millet flour to package direction. Add in all spices together and stir.

2. Reduce heat and simmer, uncovered, for 5 minutes, stirring occasionally.

3. When cooked, add sweetener to taste.

Servings: 6

Nutrition Facts (per serving)

Carbs: 11,13g

Fiber: 2,6g

154

Protein: 1,9g

Fat: 2.82g

Calories: 58,18

Scrambled Eggs with Bacon and Gouda Cheese

Ingredients

4 strips cooked bacon

4 eggs

2 1/2 Tbsp olive oil

1/4 cup softened cream cheese

1/4 cup shredded Gouda cheese

garlic and onion powder

black or white pepper

Directions

1. In a frying pan heat some olive oil and fry bacon slices until crisp .

2. In a small bowl beat the eggs with onion and garlic powder, cream cheese and Gouda shredded cheese. Season with salt and pepper to taste.

3. Pour egg mixture over bacon slices and cook for 3-4 minutes. Serve and enjoy!

Servings: 4

Cooking Time: 15 minutes

Nutrition Facts (per serving)

Carbs: 1,47g

Fiber: 0g

Protein: 14,44g

Fat: 25,94g

Calories: 380,72

Beet Cucumber Smoothie

Ingredients

1 cup spinach leaves

2 cups cucumber (peeled, seeded and chopped)

1/2 cup carrot chopped

1/2 cup fresh beetroot

3/4 cup heavy (whipping) cream

4 tsp sweetener of your choice (optional)

Handful of ground almonds

1 cup ice cubes

1 cup water

Directions

1. Place all ingredients in a blender.

2. Pulse until smooth.

3. Serve immediately.

Servings: 4

Cooking Time: 5 minutes

Nutrition Facts (per serving)

Carbs: 6,19g

Protein: 1,66g

Fat: 12.99g

Calories: 137,91

Cilantro and Ginger Smoothie

Ingredients

1/2 cup fresh cilantro (chopped)

2 inch ginger, fresh

1 cucumber

2 Tbsp chia seeds

1/2 cup spinach, fresh

1 Tbsp almond butter

Handful of ground almond

1 lime (or lemon)

2 cups water

Directions

1. Blend spinach, coriander and water until smooth.
2. Add the remaining fruits and blend again.

Servings: 3

Cooking Time: 5 minutes

Nutrition Facts (per serving)

Carbs: 11,98g

Fiber: 6,88g

Protein:

Fat: 6.92g

Calories: 102,72

Green Coconut Smoothie

Ingredients

1 cup coconut milk

1 green apple, cored and chopped

1 cup spinach

1 cucumber

2 Tbsp shaved coconut

1/2 cup water

ice cubes (if needed)

Directions

1. Put all ingredients and ice in a blender; pulse until smooth.

2. Serve immediately.

Servings: 2

Cooking Time: 5 minutes

Nutrition Facts (per serving)

Carbs: 18,11g

Fiber: 4g

Protein: 2,88g

Fat: 16,56g

Calories: 216,57

Green Devil Smoothie

Ingredients

3 cup kale, fresh

1/2 cup coconut yogurt

1/2 cup broccoli, florets

2 celery stalk, chopped

2 cup water

1 Tbsp lemon juice

ice cubes (if needed)

Directions

1. Blend all ingredients together until smooth and slightly frothy.

Servings: 2

Cooking Time: 10 minutes

Nutrition Facts (per serving)

Carbs: 16,42g

Fiber: 6,18g

Protein: 4,09g

Fat: 4,98g

Calories: 117,09

Green Dream Smoothie

Ingredients

1 cup raw cucumber, peeled and sliced

4 cups water

1 cup romaine lettuce

1 cup Haas avocado

2 Tbsp fresh basil

sweetener of your choice (optional)

handful of walnuts

2 Tbsp fresh parsley

1 Tbsp fresh ginger grated

ice cubes (optional)

Directions

1. In a blender, combine all of the ingredients and puls until smooth.

2. Add ice if used. Serve cold.

Servings: 4

Nutrition Facts (per serving)

Carbs: 4,1g

Protein: 1,1g

Fat: 3,89g

Calories: 50,62

Green Pistachio Smoothie

Ingredients

2 celery stem with leaves

1 cup spinach leaves, roughly chopped

1/2 cup pistachio nuts (unsalted)

1/2 avocado, chopped

1/2 cup lime, juice

1 Tbsp Hemp seeds

1 Tbsp soaked almonds

1 cup coconut water or water

ice cubes (optional)

Directions

1. Mix all ingredients in a blender with a few ice cubes until smooth.

Servings: 2

Cooking Time: 10 minutes

Nutrition Facts (per serving)

Carbs: 14,4g

Fiber: 9,8g

Protein: 11,08g

Fat: 17,88g

Calories: 349,55

Lime Peppermint Smoothie

Ingredients

1/4 cup fresh mint leaves

1/4 cup lime juice

1/2 cup cucumber, chopped

1 Tbsp fresh basil leaves, chopped

1 tsp chia seed (optional)

Handful of chia seeds

3 tsp zest of limes

sweetener of your choice to taste

1 cup water, divided

Ice as needed

Directions

1. Place all ingredients in a blender or food processor. Pulse until smooth well.

2. Fill glasses with ice, pour the limeade into each glass, and enjoy!

Servings: 4

Cooking Times

Total Time: 5 minutes

Nutrition Facts (per serving)

167

Carbs: 4,49g

Fiber: 1,98g

Protein: 0,84g

Fat: 1,16g

Calories: 28,11

Red Grapefruit Kale Smoothies

Ingredients

2 cups Cantaloupe

1/4 cup fresh strawberries

8 oz coconut yogurt

2 cups kale leaves, chopped

2 Tbsp sweetener of your taste

1 Ice as needed

1 cup water

Directions

1. Clean the grapefruit and remove the seeds.

2. Combine all ingredients in an electric blender and whirl until smooth. Add ice if used and serve.

Servings: 4

Cooking Time: 10 minutes

Nutrition Facts (per serving)

Carbs: 14g

Fiber: 7,23g

Protein: 4,42g

Fat: 11,57g

Calories: 260,74

Simple Avocado Smoothie

Ingredients

2.6 oz avocado

2 cup water

2 tsp chia seeds

0.5 oz fresh spinach

2 fl oz heavy whipping cream

1 tsp vanilla extract, unsweetened

1 Tbsp extra virgin coconut oil

liquid Stevia extract

few ice cubes

Directions

1. First, bisect the avocado. Carefully remove the seed.
2. In a blender, put all ingredients, sweetener and the ice (if used) and beat until smooth. Serve.

Servings: 2

Cooking Time: 10 minutes

Nutrition Facts (per serving)

Carbs: 4,46g

Protein: 1,66g

Fat: 23,63g

Calories: 226,44

Vanilla Protein Smoothie

Ingredients

1 cup baby spinach

5 Tbsp of heavy cream

3 Tbsp organic nut butter of your choice

1/2 cup vanilla protein powder

3 Tbsp sweetener of your choice

1 cup of water

Ice cubes

Directions

1. Place all ingredients in a blender and pulse until smooth well.

2. Serve with ice cubes (optional).

Servings: 2

Cooking Time: 5 minutes

Nutrition Facts (per serving)

Carbs: 11,88g

Fiber: 4,63g

Protein: 8,41g

Fat: 21,79g

Calories: 256,18

Ail Creamy Brussels Sprouts

Ingredients

10 Brussels sprouts

4 cloves garlic

1/4 cup cream cheese

2 Tbsp extra virgin olive oil

1 tsp Balsamic vinegar

salt and pepper to taste

Directions

1. Clean the Brussels Sprouts discarding the first leaves and cut into julienne strips.

2. Peel and chop the garlic cloves.

3. In a frying pan, heat the olive oil and saute the Brussels Sprouts and garlic,

4. When the garlic and sprouts are tender, turn off the heat and add the cheese. Let sit for a couple of minutes.

5. Transfer to plate and enjoy!

Servings: 1

Cooking Time: 15 minutes

Nutrition Facts (per serving)

Carbs: 16,99g

Fiber: 6,22g

Protein: 9,27g

Fat: 12,55g

Calories: 223,26

Baked Broccoli with Mushrooms and Parmesan

Ingredients

4 cups broccoli

2 cups mushrooms (chopped fine)

2 Tbsp minced garlic

1/2 tsp dried oregano

3 Tbsp grated Parmesan

salt and ground black pepper to taste

Directions

1. Preheat oven to 300F. Line a baking sheet with parchment paper.

2. Wash and slice broccoli into florets. In a bowl, toss broccoli and finely chopped mushrooms in olive oil. Season with dried oregano, salt and pepper to taste.

3. Spread all vegetables evenly over the prepared baking pan. Bake for 20-25 minutes until the broccoli is browned.

4. When done, leave to cool 5 minutes, sprinkle with Parmesan cheese and serve.

Servings: 2

Cooking Times

Total Time: 35 minutes

Nutrition Facts (per serving)

Carbs: 16,22g

Fiber: 3,33g

Protein: 12,16g

Fat: 3,51g

Calories: 138,26

Baked Buckwheat Pancakes with Hazelnuts

Ingredients

1/2 cup buckwheat flour

3 eggs

1/2 cup coconut cream

1 vanilla bean (seeds only)

1 pinch of salt

3 Tbsp olive oil

Liquid sweetener of your choice

hazelnuts

Directions

1. Preheat oven to 400F degrees.

2. Grease an oval baking pan.

3. In a large bowl, add eggs, milk, flour, vanilla and salt. Mix the ingredients until the mixture become homogeneous.

4. Pour batter in prepared oval baking pan evenly. Bake for 15-20 minutes.

5. Remove the pancake from the pan and serve with sweetener of your taste and hazelnuts.

Servings: 2

Cooking Times

Total Time: 30 minutes

Nutrition Facts (per serving)

Carbs: 17,46g

Fiber: 3g

Protein: 14,4g

Fat: 22,66g

Calories: 390,07

Baked Parmesan-Almond Zucchini

Ingredients

2 zucchinis, thinly sliced to about 1-inch thick rounds

3 large eggs, beaten

1 cup almond flour

1 cup almonds, ground

1 cup grated Parmesan cheese

1 tsp dried oregano

salt and pepper

Directions

1. Preheat oven to 400 F degrees. Line a large baking sheet with parchment paper.

2. Wash, clean and slice zucchinis. Salt from all sides and let dry on a paper towel. Set aside.

3. In a plate, combine ground almond, Parmesan cheese, oregano and season with salt and pepper to taste and oregano; set aside.

4. In another shallow plate add the almond flour.

5. In a third plate beat eggs, with salt and pepper.

6. Start dredging zucchini rounds in flour, dip into eggs, then dredge in almond mixture, pressing to coat. Place zucchini slices on prepared baking sheet.

7. Bake for 20 to 30 minutes, or until the zucchini rounds are golden and crispy.

8. Serve hot.

Servings: 6

Cooking Times

Preparation Time: 15 minutes

Cooking Time: 25 minutes

Nutrition Facts (per serving)

Carbs: 16,36g

Dietary Fiber: 3,28g

Protein: 12,12g

Fat: 17,49g

Calories: 288

Double Cheese Artichoke Dip

Ingredients

2 cup artichoke hearts, chopped

16 oz shredded Mozzarella cheese

1 cup grated Parmesan cheese

1 cup heavy (whipping) cream

1 cup green onion, grated

Directions

1. Mix all ingredients together and put in a Slow Cooker.
2. Cook on HIGH mode for about one hour.
3. Sprinkle with chopped green onion, if desired.

Servings: 12

Cooking Times

Total Time: 1 hour

Nutrition Facts (per serving)

Carbs: 10,44g

Fiber: 1,74g

Protein: 13,67g

Total Fat: 15g

Calories: 227

Easy Slow Cooker Artichokes

Ingredients

4 artichokes

3 Tbsp lemon juice

2 Tbsp coconut butter, melted

1 tsp salt and ground black pepper to taste

water

Directions

1. Wash and trim artichokes.

2. Start by pulling off the outermost leaves until you get down to the lighter yellow leaves.

3. Then, using a serrated knife, cut off the top third or so of the artichoke.

4. With the same serrated knife, trim the very bottom of the stem.

5. Mix together salt, melted coconut butter and lemon juice and pour over artichokes.

6. Pour in water to cover 3 of artichokes. Cover and cook on LOW 8-10 hours or on HIGH 2-4 hours.

7. Serve and enjoy!

Servings: 4

Cooking Times

Total Time: 2 hours and 10 minutes

Nutrition Facts (per serving)

Carbs: 14,52g

Fiber: 6,95g

Protein: 4,29g

Fat: 6,98g

Calories: 113

Eggs with Motley Peppers and Zucchini

Ingredients

6 eggs

2 zucchini, diced

1 spring onion, chopped

1 green pepper, finely diced

1 yellow pepper, finely diced

1 red pepper, finely diced

3 Tbsp coconut oil (melted)

salt and fresh ground black pepper to taste

Directions

1. In a non-stick frying skillet, heat 2 Tbsp olive oil in a pan and sauté the onion for 5 minutes.

2. Add the peppers and fry for 2-3 minutes more.

3. Next, add the zucchini and sauté for another 3 minutes. Remove from heat and set aside.

4. In a medium bowl beat the eggs with salt.

5. Mix the vegetables into the eggs.

6. Heat the remaining olive oil in the frying pan and pour in the egg and vegetable mixture.

7. Cook for 2-3 minutes constantly stirring.

8. Serve hot.

Servings: 4

Cooking Times

185

Total Time: 25 minutes

Nutrition Facts (per serving)

Carbs: 12,77g

Fiber: 3,26g

Protein: 12,04g

Fat: 7.94g

Calories: 165

Electric Pressure Cooker Bok Choy Salad

Ingredients

1 bunch bok choi, trimmed

1 cup or more water

Salt

Olive oil

Lime

Directions

1. Place the stems in your Electric pressure cooker and pour one cup, or more water to just-cover the stems.

2. Close and lock the lid of the pressure cooker. Turn the heat up to high and when the cooker reaches pressure, lower to the heat to the minimum required by the cooker to maintain pressure.

3. Cook for 5-7 minutes at high pressure.

4. When time is up, open the cooker by Slow releasing the pressure.

5. Pull out the leaves and stems with tongs, and put on a small serving plate.

6. Dress with salt and olive oil before serving. Sprinkle some lime juice.

Servings: 3

Cooking Times

Total Time: 10 minutes

Nutrition Facts (per serving)

Carbs: 6,1g

Fiber: 2,8g

Protein: 4,2g

Fat: 0,56g

Calories: 36,4

Kale, Peppers and Crumbled Feta Omelet (Slow Cooker)

Ingredients

8 eggs, well beaten

1 cup red peppers, diced

1/4 cup green onions (finely chopped)

1/2 cup crumbled Feta

3/4 cup kale, chopped

2 tsp olive oil

1/2 tsp Italian seasoning

Salt and freshly ground pepper, to taste

sour cream cheese or cottage (optional)

Directions

1. In a large frying pan heat oil on medium-high. Add chopped kale and cook about 3-4 minutes.

2. Wash and chop the red peppers. Slice the green onions and crumble the Feta. Grease the bottom of your Slow Cooker with olive oil. Add the chopped red pepper and sliced green onion to Slow Cooker with the kale.

3. In a small bowl, beat the eggs and pour over other ingredients in Slow Cooker. Stir well and add Italian seasonings. Adjust salt and pepper to taste.

4. Cook on LOW for 2 - 3 hours. Serve hot, with a dollop of sour cream if desired.

Servings: 4

Cooking Times

Total Time: 3 hours

Nutrition Facts (per serving)

Carbs: 4,56g

Fiber: 1,01g

Protein: 11,78g

Fat: 23,87g

Calories: 279,34

Atkins Almond Buns

Ingredients

3 almond flour

5 Tbs butter, unsalted

2 eggs

1.5 tsp sweetener of your choice (optional)

1.5 tsp baking powder

Directions

1. Preheat oven to 350F.

2. Combine the dry ingredients in a bowl.

3. In a separate bowl, whisk the eggs.

4. Melt butter, add to mixture and whisk well.

5. Divide mixture equally into 6 parts and place in a greased baking dish.

6. Bake for 12-15 minutes.

7. Let cool on a wire rack.

Servings: 3

Cooking Time: 20 minutes

Nutrition Facts (per serving)

Carbs: 2,44g

Fiber: 0,2g

Protein: 4,45g

Fat: 22,43g

Calories: 225,58

Mini Ham Omelets Muffins

Ingredients

11 oz Ham Steak

10 green onions Green Onions

12 Eggs

1/2 cup of Heavy cream

9 slices mushrooms

9 Slices Cheddar Cheese

coconut oil for greasing

Salt, Pepper, Onion Powder, Garlic Powder to taste

Directions

1. Preheat oven to 350F. Grease the muffin pan with coconut oil.
2. Dice the ham steak, slice the green onions and wash the mushrooms.
3. In a deep bowl, beat the eggs. Add in the heavy cream and spices along with ham cubes and sliced green onions.
4. Adjust salt, pepper and spices to taste.
5. Fill each cavity of muffin pan with the egg mixture.
6. Bake in oven for 4-5 minutes.
7. Remove from the oven and add the mushrooms on the top
8. Cook for 8-9 more minutes or until the eggs are mostly set.
9. Add Cheddar cheese and cook for 1 more minute.
10. Serve hot.

Servings: 18

Cooking Times

Total Time: 25 minutes

Nutrition Facts (per serving)

Carbs: 1,54g

Fiber: 0,32g

Protein: 11,69g

Fat: 11,1g

Calories: 153,55

Nonpareil Bacon Waffles

Ingredients

4 slices bacon

2 eggs

3 cup almond flour

5 Tbsp melted butter or ghee

1.5 tsp baking powder

1.5 tsp sweetener of your choice

Directions

1. Microwave the butter and set aside.

2. In a frying pan, cook the bacon until crisp.

3. First, mix the dry ingredients first (almond flour, baking powder and sweetener of your choice)

4. Add the two eggs and mix thoroughly. Add the melted butter and mix.

5. Preheat the waffle maker.

6. When it is preheated, open it, fill with batter and place 2 slices of bacon over top.

7. Close and flip the waffle maker, when it beeps, flip it over and remove the waffle with a fork.

8. Serve hot.

Servings: 2

Cooking Times

Total Time: 15 minutes

Nutrition Facts (per serving)

Carbs: 5,1g

Fiber: 2,65g

Protein: 8,35g

Fat: 24,97g

Calories: 323,24

Power Greens and Sausage Casserole

Ingredients

12 eggs

1 1/4 lbs chicken or turkey sausage

1 cup kale leaves, chopped

1 cup arugula leaves, chopped

2 cups spinach, finely chopped

2 small zucchini - peeled

1 green onion, chopped

1/4 cup coconut milk

1/2 Tbsp coconut oil

1 tsp garlic powder

1 tsp sea salt

1 tsp pepper

Directions

1. Heat oven to 365 degrees. Grease casserole dish with coconut oil.

2. In a frying pan, melt coconut oil over medium heat, Add in sausage and stir with a wooden spoon. Cook for two to three minutes.

3. In a big bowl beat eggs.

4. Chop the green onion and peeled the zucchini. Mix into eggs with seasoning, all greens and coconut milk.

5. Pour in egg mixture and stir in sausage. Adjust the salt and pepper to taste. Cook for 45 minutes.

6. Cover with foil and cook for 10-15 minutes more.
    7. Serve hot.

Servings: 10

Cooking Times

Total Time: 20 minutes

Nutrition Facts (per serving)

Carbs: 11,88g

Fiber: 1,48g

Protein: 12,19g

Fat: 7,98g

Calories: 165,48

Radish, Bacon and Egg Scramble

Ingredients

6 oz radishes

4 oz Cheddar cheese

8 oz flank steak

2 oz bacon

4 eggs

Salt and Pepper to taste

Directions

1. Preheat oven to 450 degrees F. Wash the radishes, then cut the ends and quarter. Set aside.

2. In a frying pan, cook the flank steak for 5 minutes flipping from one side to another.

3. Pan fry the radishes and bacon in a cast iron skillet for about 5-6 minutes or until the radishes turn golden brown

4. Slice the flank steak and add into the pan.

5. Add the cheese and break the eggs into the mixture, season to taste and cook for one to two minutes.

6. Transfer to the oven and cook for 12 minutes until the eggs are set to the desired leve.

7. Serve and enjoy!

Servings: 4

Cooking Times

Total Time: 25 minutes

Nutrition Facts (per serving)

Carbs: 2,26g

Fiber: 0,68g

Protein: 27,42g

Fat: 22,04g

Calories: 348,58

Sautéed Cabbage and Brussels Sprouts (Electric Pressure Cooker)

Ingredients

4 medium beets

1-1/2 lbs cabbage, cut into wedges

1-1/2 lbs Brussels sprouts

8 large cloves garlic, left unpeeled

3 Tbsp olive oil

1 Tbsp chopped fresh thyme

1/2 tsp salt, plus more to taste

1/4 tsp freshly ground black pepper

Directions

1. In your Electric Pressure Cooker add chopped vegetables, oil, salt and freshly ground black pepper.

2. Select SAUTE and cook under HIGH pressure for 15 minutes.

3. When ready, select natural release. Carefully open the lid.

4. Transfer all vegetables from the cooker to the serving plate, toss well and serve.

Servings: 6

Cooking Times

Total Time: 15 minutes

Nutrition Facts (per serving)

Total Carbs: 16,11g

Fiber: 6,57g

Protein: 6,2g

Fat: 8,31g

Calories: 160,91

Simple Bacon Pepper Pot

Ingredients

6 slices bacon

4 Eggs

1 small green pepper

Jalapeno pepper, sliced

1 green onion

Directions

1. Slice the pepper, green onion and jalapeno into thin strips.
2. In a frying pan, cook the vegetables about 2-3 minutes until browned.
3. Chop the bacon in a food processor until it breaks into chunks.
4. Mix all the ingredients together.
5. Cook the hash until the bacon is approaching crisp.
6. Arrange on a plate and top with a fried egg!
7. Serve and enjoy!

Servings: 2

Cooking Time: 25 minutes

Nutrition Facts (per serving)

Carbs: 4,41g

Fiber: 1,44g

Protein: 23,33g

Fat: 29,87g

Calories: 499

Sour and Spicy Goat Skewers

Ingredients

1 lb boneless goat loin, cut into cubes

2 Tbsp lime juice (freshly squeezed)

1 cup coconut yogurt

1/4 tsp ground ginger

3/4 tsp turmeric

1/2 tsp ground cumin

1 Tbs ground coriander

1/2 tsp salt

Skewers

Directions

1. In a medium bowl, stir together coconut yogurt, lime juice and all seasonings; mix well.

2. Add the goat meat cubes to the bowl, stir to coat with the marinade, cover and refrigerate for 6-8 hours.

3. Remove the meat from the marinade, pat lightly with paper towels to dry.

4. Place meat evenly on the skewers. Grill over medium-hot coals, turning frequently, for about 10 minutes until nicely brown.

5. Serve and enjoy without guilty.

Servings: 2

Cooking Times

Inactive Time: 10 minutes

Total Time: 25 minutes

Nutrition Facts (per serving)

Carbs: 12,24g

Fiber: 1,25g

Protein: 26,77g

Fat: 9,79g

Calories: 342,93

Sour Sausages with Shallots and Kalamata Olives

Ingredients

1 lb sausages chopped

4 shallots, finely chopped

1/2 cup lemon juice (2 lemons)

16 black and green Kalamata olives

2 Tbsp whole grain mustard

4 Tbsp extra virgin olive oil

salt and ground black pepper to taste

Directions

1. Preheat oven to 400F. Grease an roasting pan and place in the sausages and chopped shallots.
2. Roast for 20 minutest.
3. When ready, remove the meat from the sausages and season with salt and freshly ground pepper to taste
4. Pour the lemon juice into the roasting tin.
5. Add in the mustard and chopped olives and simmer gently for 2-3 minutes. Pour lemon mixture over the sausages and shallots.
6. Place on serving plate and serve.

Servings: 6

Cooking Times

Total Time: 30 minutes

Nutrition Facts (per serving)

Carbs: 14,9g

Fiber: 0,42g

Protein: 18,48

Fat: 16,67g

Calories: 408

Spinach and Cheese Stuffed Mushrooms

Ingredients

12 large mushroom caps with stems

1 cream cheese

1 cup cooked, chopped spinach

1 Tbsp garlic, minced

1 tsp red pepper flakes

2 scallions, finely chopped

1 tsp salt

1 tsp fresh cracked pepper

3 tsp extra virgin olive oil

2 Tbsp almond, ground

2 Tbsp Parmesan cheese

1 tsp granulated garlic

1 Tbsp fresh flat leaf parsley, finely chopped

Directions

1. Preheat the oven to 400 degrees F.
2. First, remove the mushrooms stems. Chop the stems finely.
3. Heat a frying skillet with 2 teaspoons of olive oil and cook the mushrooms stems for 5 minutes.
4. In a bowl, combine the cream cheese, red pepper flakes, scallions, chopped spinach, minced garlic, cooked mushroom stems, salt and pepper.
5. In a small bowl, combine ground almonds, parmesan cheese, parsley and granulated garlic.
6. Fill the mushroom cavities with cheese and mushrooms mixture. Sprinkle the ground almonds mixture over each mushroom.

7. Drizzle the remaining 1 teaspoon of oil over the filling in the mushroom caps.

8. Bake in oven about 12 minutes.

9. Serve hot.

Servings: 6

Cooking Times

Preparation Time: 8 minutes

Cooking Time: 12 minutes

Total Time: 20 minutes

Nutrition Facts (per serving)

Carbs: 11,36g

Fiber: 5,24g

Protein: 11,75g

Fat: 6,36g

Calories: 138,32

Spinach-Chard Puree with Almonds

Ingredients

1 lb baby spinach leaves

1/2 lb Swiss chard, tough stems removed, tender stems and leaves torn into 2" pieces

1 cup cauliflower flowerets (1 cup)

1 leek

1/4 cup extra virgin olive oil

3 cups water

4 Tbsp toasted almond slivers

1/4 cup tofu cheese, cubed

salt and black ground pepper to taste

Directions

1. Wash the leek and cut it into thick slices.
2. Heat the olive oil in a saucepan and cook the leek and cauliflower for about 2-3 minutes.
3. Add the chard and cleaned spinach leaves, water and a pinch of salt and pepper to taste. Bring to the boil and let it simmer for 15 minutes.
4. Remove from the heat and place the vegetables in a food processor. Blend into a very smooth soup.
5. Pour the mixture into bowls, place some tofu cubes on top and generously sprinkle with ground toasted almonds.

Servings: 10

Cooking Times

211

Total Time: 35 minutes

Nutrition Facts (per serving)

Carbs: 6,92g

Fiber: 1,88g

Protein: 5,24g

Fat: 1,69g

Calories: 47,47

Delish Hash

Ingredients

1 pc. medium-sized zucchini, diced

2 bacon strips, sliced

½ onion, chopped

1 tbsp. ghee

1 tbsp. fresh parsley, chopped

salt to taste

Directions

1. Heat the ghee on a pan over medium heat. Add the chopped onions and bacon slices into the pan and cook for a few minutes to allow the onions to sweat. Stir frequently.

2. Throw the diced zucchini into the pan and cook for another 12-15 minutes.

3. Transfer the hash into a pan, season with salt and garnish with chopped fresh parsley on top.

4. Serve with scrambled egg on the side.

Serves 1

Nutritional Information

Calories 54

Net Carbs 1.4g

Fats 4.2g

Protein 2.9g

Fiber 3.0 g

Fisherman's Breakfast

Ingredients

2 organic eggs

1 small jar sardines in olive oil

2 tbsp. artichoke hearts, cut into wedges

½ cup arugula

salt and pepper to taste

Directions

1. Set oven at 375F

2. Lay the sardines on an oven-proof dish. Break the eggs on top and then top again with the arugula leaves and artichokes.

3. Season with salt and pepper.

4. Place in the oven to cook for 10 minutes or until the eggs are cooked through.

5. Serve hot.

Serves 1

Nutritional Information

Calories 245

Net Carbs 1.1g

Fats 15.2g

Protein 25.1g

Fiber 0g

Herbed Eggs

Ingredients

4 eggs

2 cloves of garlic, minced

1 tsp. fresh thyme

½ fresh parsley, chopped

½ cup fresh cilantro, chopped

¼ tsp. cayenne pepper, ground

¼ tsp. cumin, ground

salt to taste

2 tbsp. organic butter

Directions

1. Heat the butter on a non-stick pan over low heat.

2. Add the minced garlic into the hot pan and sauté for 3 minutes. Add the fresh thyme into the pan and cook for another half a minute.

3. Throw in the chopped parsley and cilantro, stir, and cook for another 3 minutes.

4. Carefully crack the eggs directly to the pan and cover. Add the seasonings.

5. Cook the eggs for 5-6 minutes depending on your preferred doneness.

6. Serve with sausages or bacon on the side.

Serves 2

Nutritional Information

Calories 299

Net Carbs 3.2g

Fats 27.3g

Protein 12.0g

Fiber 0.9g

Smoked Salmon and Avocado Breakfast Salad

Ingredients

1 pc. ripe avocado, peel removed and cut into cubes

¼ cup smoked salmon

2 tbsp. softened goat cheese

2 tbsp. ghee

2 tbsp. lemon juice

salt to taste

Directions

1. Cut the avocado into cubes and place in serving bowl.

2. Add the smoked salmon and carefully toss together.

3. Add the rest of the ingredients and combine.

4. Season with salt before serving.

Serves 1-2

Nutritional Information

Calories 366

Net Carbs 9.1g

Fats 35.1g

Protein 7.6g

Fiber 6.8g

Creamy Greens Breakfast Pie

Ingredients

1 lb. sausage

8 cups baby spinach

3 organic eggs

1 cup mozzarella, shredded

2 cups ricotta cheese

¼ cup parmesan cheese, shredded

1 tbsp. organic butter

1 clove of garlic, minced

1 small onion, chopped

1/8 tsp. nutmeg, ground

salt and pepper

Directions

1. Set the oven at 350F.

2. Heat the butter on a pan over medium heat. Sauté the onion and garlic for 3-4 minutes.

3. Add the baby spinach into the pan and cook for another 5 minutes or until the leaves wilt.

4. Season with nutmeg, salt and pepper. Stir and turn off the heat. Set aside.

5. Beat the eggs in a large bowl and whisk in all the cheeses. Mix well.

6. Add the cooked greens in the bowl with the eggs and combine.

7. Meanwhile, place the sausage into a baking dish, press, and mold it into a pie crust.

8. Pour the egg and spinach mixture into the pie crust and place in the oven to cook for 35 minutes, or until the eggs are firm.

Remember to place a baking sheet below the baking dish so you do not end up with a messy oven!

Serves 4-5

Nutritional Information

Calories 584

Net Carbs 9.4g

Fats 42.7g

Protein 40.2g

Fiber 1.4g

Atkins Breakfast Biscuit

Ingredients

2 large eggs, (separate the white and yolk of one egg)

¼ cup softened cream cheese

2 tbsp. parmesan cheese, grated

½ tsp. psyllium husks

½ tsp. organic apple cider vinegar

a pinch of baking powder

a pinch of garlic powder

salt and pepper to taste

1 tsp. olive oil, plus ½ tsp. for cooking

1 slice of American cheese cut in half

Directions

1. In a bowl, whisk together the egg white from one egg, cream cheese, parmesan, psyllium husk, apple cider, baking powder, and garlic powder. Combine well.

2. Brush 2 ramekins with the olive oil and pour the prepared batter. Place in the microwave to cook for 35 seconds on high.

3. Heat the left over oil on a non-stick pan and add the remaining eggs and fry until over medium.

4. Place the cheese slices and fried eggs on top of the cooked biscuits and serve immediately.

Serves 2

Nutritional Information

Calories 68

Net Carbs 4.3g

Fats 9.9

Protein 8.3g

Fiber 2.4g

Delicious Sausage Biscuits

Ingredients

½ cup softened cream cheese

1 organic egg

2 cloves of garlic, minced

1 tbsp. chives, chopped

salt to taste

½ tsp. Italian seasoning

1 cup sharp cheddar cheese, shredded

¼ cup heavy cream

1 ½ cup almond flour

¼ cup water

½ lb. cooked ground sausage

Directions

1. Set the oven at 350F

2. In a bowl, combine together and whip the softened cream cheese and eggs using a hand mixer. Add the minced garlic, chives, salt, and Italian seasoning into the bowl and carefully mix.

3. Also add in the cheddar, heavy cream, almond, flour, and water into the mix. And combine well.

4. Take the cooked ground sausage and gradually add it in the cream cheese mixture.

5. Prepare a muffin pan by greasing it with oil or butter and then fill the muffin cups (about 8) with the prepared mixture.

6. Place in the oven to bake at 25 minutes.

7. Allow the biscuits to cook before removing from the pan and serving.

Serves 4

Nutritional Information

Calories 437

Net Carbs 2.3g

Fats 37.7g

Protein 21.9g

Fiber 0g

All-in Frittatas

Ingredients

½ cup cooked ground sausage

2 cups yellow bell pepper, diced

10 organic eggs

2 egg whites

½ cup milk

½ tsp. salt

½ tbsp. butter

pepper to taste

½ cup pepper jack cheese, shredded

green onions, chopped for garnish

Directions

1. Set oven at 350F.

2. Melt the butter in a non-stick pan heated over medium-high fire.

3. Add the bell peppers in the hot pan and cook until it softens. Set aside

4. In a bowl, whisk together the whole eggs, egg whites, and milk.

5. Divide the cooked ground sausage on 12 muffin tins and then top with the cooked bell peppers.

6. Evenly pour the egg mixture into the tins and season with salt and pepper.

7. Sprinkle with generous amounts of pepper jack cheese on top and then carefully stir the ingredients in the tins using a fork.

8. Place in the oven to cook for 25 minutes, or until the egg is cooked through.

9. Garnish with the chopped green onions on top.

Serves 6

Nutritional Information

Calories 152

Net Carbs 4.2g

Fats 9.4g

Protein 13.7g

Fiber 0.8g

Olives and Avocado Frittata

Ingredients

4 organic eggs cut into thick slices

1 ripe avocado

10 pcs. pitted olives

½ cup brie cheese, sliced thin

1 tsp. Italian seasoning

2 tbsp. ghee

2 tbsp. olive oil

salt to taste

Directions

1. In a large mixing bowl, whisk together the eggs, olives, Italian seasoning, and salt. Whisk until frothy. Set aside.

2. In a non-stick skillet, add the ghee and heat over medium fire. Add the avocado slices into the hot pan and fry until the avocadoes turn golden brown. Set aside.

3. Using the same pan, increase the heat to high and pour in the egg mixture.

4. Add the brie cheese into the pan, cover and cook for 3 minutes.

5. Flip the frittata and cook for another 2-3 minutes.

6. Serve the frittata with the fried avocadoes on top.

Makes 2

Nutritional Information

227

Calories 690

Net Carbs 9.7g

Fats 65.7g

Protein 20.5g

Fiber 6.7g

Cheesy Cauli Waffle

Ingredients

¾ cup cauliflower florets

2 organic eggs

¼ cup cheddar

¼ cup mozzarella

1 tbsp. chives

¼ tsp. onion powder

¼ tsp. garlic powder

salt and pepper to taste

Directions

1. Place the cauliflower, cheddar, and mozzarella in a food processor and pulse until all the ingredients are chopped and mixed.

2. Add the eggs and the rest of the ingredients into the food processor and blend. Make sure that the ingredients are well-combined.

3. Heat your waffle maker and pour the mixture in it to cook based on the product instructions.

4. Serve the waffle warm with cream cheese and bacon on the side

Makes 2

Nutritional Information

Calories 140

Net Carbs 3.7g

Fats 7.9g

Protein 13.9g

Fiber 1g

Eggs n' Steak Breakfast

Ingredients

2 lbs. beef chuck shoulder

7 organic eggs

1 small onion, chopped

1 bell pepper, chopped

¼ cup cheddar cheese, shredded

½ heavy cream

½ tsp. garlic powder

salt and pepper to taste

½ tbsp. butter

Directions

1. Melt the butter in a pan over medium heat. Add the onion and bell peppers and cook for 4-5 minutes. Set aside.

2. Place the same pan back on the stove and increase the heat to high. Add the steaks into the pan and cook for 6 minutes on each side. Set the steaks aside to rest.

3. In a large bowl, mix together the eggs, heavy cream, garlic powder, salt and pepper.

4. Cook the egg mixture into a hot non-stick pan and stir occasionally.

5. Transfer the cooked eggs into a serving plate and serve with the sliced steaks on the side.

Serves 5

Nutritional Information

Calories 506

Net Carbs 4g

Fats 51g

Protein 45g

Fiber 1g

Bacon Hash and Eggs

Ingredients

4 organic eggs

6 bacon strips, cooked

1 onion, chopped

1 green bell pepper, chopped

1 tbsp. jalapenos, diced

1 tbsp. ghee

Directions

1. Heat the ghee in a cast iron skillet over medium heat. Add the chopped onions, bell pepper, and jalapenos, and sauté until the onions become translucent. Set aside.

2. Chop the cooked the bacon and mix into the cooked vegetables.

3. Place egg rings into a pan with oil and then scoop the veggie and bacon mixture into the rings.

4. Cook until the hash is almost crispy. Set aside

5. Fry the eggs in a pan and serve on top of the bacon hash.

Serves 2

Nutritional Information

Calories 366

Net Carbs 11g

Fats 24g

Protein 23g

Fiber 2g

Bacon Waffles

Ingredients

4 bacon strips, cooked crispy chopped

2 organic eggs

5 tbsp. melted organic butter

¾ almond flour

1 ½ tsp. stevia

1 ½ tsp. baking powder

whipped cream (as topping)

Directions

1. In a bowl, combine the flour, stevia, and baking powder together.
2. Crack the eggs into the bowl and combine well.
3. Pour in the melted butter and mix again. Set aside.
4. Heat your waffle maker and set it on medium.
5. Grease the waffle maker before pouring in the batter.
6. Sprinkle the bacon crisps on top and then cook according to equipment instructions.
7. Serve with whipped cream on top.

Serving 2

Nutritional Information

Calories 648

Net Carbs 10g

Fats 61g

Protein 21g

Fiber 5g

Ham and Cheese Omelet

Ingredients

150g ham, diced

6 organic eggs

½ cup heavy cream

¼ tsp. pepper

¼ tsp. salt

¼ tsp. garlic powder

½ cup diced tomatoes

6 pcs. green onions, chopped

4 slices cheddar cheese

Directions

1. Set the oven 350F.

2. In a large bowl, combine the eggs, heavy cream, and season with salt, pepper, and garlic powder. Add the diced ham and tomatoes, stir well.

3. Pour egg mixture in a greased muffin tin.

4. Place in the oven to cook for 5 minutes.

5. Remove the tin from the oven and then add the green onions on top.

6. Place in the oven to cook for another 8 minutes.

7. Remove again from the oven and place the cheese slices on top, and bake again for another minute.

8. Serve warm.

Makes 4

Nutritional Information

Calories 257

Net Carbs 4g

Fats 18g

Protein 17g

Fiber 1g

All-Meat Bagels

Ingredients

3 small onions, minced

2 tbsp. organic butter

4 lb. ground pork

4 organic eggs

1 ¼ cup all-natural tomato sauce

2 tsp. paprika

salt and pepper to taste

Directions

1. Set the oven at 400F.

2. Mel the butter in a non-stick pan over medium heat. Add the minced onions and sauté for a few minutes until the onions turn translucent. Set aside

3. In a large bowl, combine the ground pork, eggs, and tomato sauce. Season with salt, pepper, paprika and then add the sautéed onions.

4. Combine the ingredients using your hands and then form into 12 balls.

5. Flatten the middle of the ball to make it look like a bagel and then place on top of a baking sheet lined with parchment paper.

6. Bake in the oven to bake for 40 minutes or until cooked through.

Serves 2

Nutritional Information

Calories 805

Net Carbs 9.9g

Fats 26.4g

Protein 126g

Fiber 2.7g

Egg-Stuffed Meat Balls

Ingredients

4 organic eggs, cooked hard boiled

12oz. ground pork sausage

8 bacon slices

Directions

1. Divide the ground sausage into four and form into patties.

2. Place the hardboiled egg in the middle of the patties (one each), and cover the egg with the ground pork.

3. Place in the fridge to chill for at least 30 minutes.

4. Set oven at 450F.

5. Take 2 bacon slices and wrap around the meatballs and secure with toothpicks.

6. Place on a baking sheet and bake in the oven to cook for 20 minutes or until the bacon is crisp.

7. Serve immediately.

Serves 4

Nutritional Information

Calories 351

Net Carbs 0.3g

Fats 28.5g

Protein 22.1g

Fiber 0g

Cheeseburger Quiche

Ingredients

4 organic eggs

¼ lb. bacon

½ lb. ground beef

1 onion, chopped

½ cup mayonnaise

½ cup heavy cream

2 cups sharp cheddar cheese, shredded

salt and pepper to taste

Directions

1. Set the oven at 350F

2. Cook the bacon to a crisp and set aside

3. Using the same pan, sauté the onions, add ground beef and cook until done.

4. Meanwhile, combine the eggs, mayonnaise, and heavy cream in a bowl. Season with salt and pepper; mix well.

5. Chop the cooked bacon and add into the bowl.

6. Also add the cooked ground beef and mix well.

7. Add half of the cheese in the mixture and stir again.

8. Pour the meat and egg mixture into a baking dish into a greased baking dish, top with the rest of the cheese, and place in the oven to bake for 30 minutes or until the eggs are cooked through.

9. Allow to cool for at least 10 minutes before serving.

Makes 8

Nutritional Information

Calories 532

Net Carbs 5g

Fats 44g

Protein 27g

Fiber 0g

Hot n' Spicy Egg Scramble

Ingredients

1 green bell pepper, chopped

1 onion, chopped

1 cup cooked ham, diced

1 cup pepper jack cheese, shredded

8 organic eggs

½ tsp. chili powder

1 tsp. Sriracha sauce

¼ cup coconut milk

salt and pepper to taste

2 tbsp. ghee

Directions

1. Heat the ghee in a non-stick pan over medium fire.

2. Add the onions and bell pepper into the pan and sauté for a 5 minutes.

3. Season with salt and pepper and add the diced ham into the pan.

4. Meanwhile, in a large bowl, whisk together the eggs, chili powder, Sriracha sauce, and coconut milk.

5. Gradually add the shredded cheese into the bowl with eggs. Set aside.

6. Reduce the heat to low and then pour the egg mixture into the pan with the bell peppers and cook for 2 minutes. 40

7. Flip and then cook again until the eggs are done.

8.   Serve.

Serves 4

Nutritional Information

Calories 545

Net Carbs 10g

Fats 53.6g

Protein 35g

Fiber 0g

Chorizo Stuffed Bell Peppers

Ingredients

3 large bell peppers, cut in half, core and seeds removed

½ lb. spicy chorizo sausage, crumbled

2 cloves of garlic

1 onion, chopped

6 organic eggs

¼ cup almond milk, unsweetened

1 cup cheddar cheese, shredded

½ tbsp. ghee

salt and pepper to taste

Directions

1. Set oven at 350F

2. Heat the ghee in a non-stick pan over medium heat and cook the chorizo crumbles. Set aside

3. Using the same pan, add the onions and garlic and sauté for a few minutes. Turn off the heat and set aside.

4. In a bowl, stir together the eggs, milk, cheddar, and season with salt and pepper.

5. Add the chorizo into the bowl with the eggs and stir well.

6. Place the bell pepper halves in an oven-safe dish filled with ¼ inch of water.

7. Scoop the chorizo and egg mixture into the bell peppers and place the dish into the oven to bake for 35 minutes.

8. Serve warm.

Serves 2-3

Nutritional Information

Calories 631

Net Carbs 13g

Fats 46g

Protein 44g

Fiber 3.5g

Veggie Tofu Scramble

Ingredients

2 tbsp. olive oil

2 cloves of garlic, chopped

1 onion, chopped

½ lb. firm tofu, remove excess liquid and chop into cubes

¼ tsp. cinnamon, ground

1 tbsp. chili powder

salt and pepper to taste

1 tsp. organic apple cider vinegar

2 tbsp. fresh cilantro, chopped

Directions

1. Heat the olive oil in a non-stick pan and sauté the onions and garlic for 3-5 minutes.

2. Add the tofu into the pan and crumble.

3. Stir the tofu with the onion and garlic and season with cinnamon, chili powder, salt, and pepper.

4. Cook for 15-20 minutes, or until the tofu is done.

5. Turn off the heat and immediately add the apple cider.

6. Place the tofu scramble into serving bowls and garnish with chopped cilantro.

Serves 2

Nutritional Information

Calories 239

Net Carbs 10.4g

Fats 19.5g

Protein 10.6g

Fiber 3.7g

Atkins Bread Pudding

Ingredients

4 slices of the Protein Loaded bread,
chopped into small bites

2 organic eggs

2 tbsp. heavy cream

2 tbsp. stevia

1 tsp. cinnamon, ground

1 tbsp. organic butter

Directions

1. Set oven at 350F

2. In a bowl whisk the eggs with heavy cream and stevia.

3. Place the chopped bread into an oven-safe dish and pour over the egg mixture. Sprinkle with cinnamon.

4. Bake in the oven for 15 minutes or until the pudding has set.

5. Allow to cool before serving warm.

Serves 2

Nutritional Information

Calories 536

Net Carbs 8g

Fats 49g

Protein 18g

Avocado Breakfast Mousse

Ingredients

2 ripe avocados

1/3 cup cocoa powder

½ tsp. chia seeds

1 tsp. vanilla extract

10 drops stevia

3 tbsp. coconut oil

Directions

1. Place all the ingredients in a blender and blend until smooth.
2. Pour the mixture into a bowl and place in the fridge to chill for 40 minutes or more.
3. Serve chilled.

Serves 2

Nutritional Information

Calories 462

Net Carbs 15g

Fats 46g

Protein 6g

Fiber 1.2g

Bacon and Peanut Butter Muffin Cups

Ingredients

2 tbsp. all-natural peanut butter

2 bacon strips, cooked and chopped

1 cup almond flour

1 tsp. baking powder

1 organic egg

2 tbsp. heavy cream

1 tsp. vanilla extract

Directions

1. Set oven at 350F

2. In a bowl, mix together the almond flour and baking powder.

3. Beat the egg lightly and add into the dry ingredients.

4. Also add the heavy cream, vanilla extract, chopped bacon, and all-natural peanut butter. Stir well.

5. Pour the batter into greased muffin tins and place in the oven to bake for 15 minutes or until the toothpick comes out clean after being inserted in to the muffins.

6. Serve warm.

Serves 4

Nutritional Information

Calories 270

Net Carbs 8g

Fats 23g

Protein 10g

Power Green Fuel

Ingredients

1 cup almond milk, unsweetened

1 cup baby spinach

½ ripe avocado

½ tbsp. stevia

1 cup ice

Directions

1. Place all the ingredients into a blender and blend until smooth.

2. Serve and consume immediately.

Serves 1

Nutritional Information

Calories 382

Net Carbs 11.5g

Fats 38.5g

Protein 4.1g

Fiber 6.3g

Lunch Recipes

Baked Creamy Cauliflower-Broccoli Chicken

Ingredients

2 boneless chicken breasts

1 cup chicken broth

3 cups cauliflower

3 cups broccoli, steamed and chopped

2 cups shredded Cheddar cheese

1 cup heavy cream

1 small yellow onion

1/2 Tbsp. minced garlic

1 tsp. lemon juice

1/2 cup mayonnaise

3 Tbsp. ghee

fresh parsley, chopped

salt and fresh pepper to taste

Directions

1. Preheat the oven to 350 degrees.

2. In a deep saucepot boil chicken breast until the chicken is cooked through.

3. Meanwhile, in a frying pan with the ghee cook up the garlic and onions on a low heat. Add all spices one by one stirring frequently.

4. While that's cooking, in a food processor blend up your cauliflower.

5. When the onions are soft, add the cauliflower. Cook for 2-3 minutes. Add in the chicken broth. Cook, covered for about 10 minutes.

6. Add the heavy cream and lemon juice and let simmer uncovered on low for about 10 minutes more. At the end, add in mayonnaise and stir.

7. Pull apart your chicken and add half of chicken into the cauliflower cream mixture.

8. Use the other half to line the bottom of an 8x8 casserole dish. On top of the chicken, layer in chopped broccoli.

9. Top with the cauliflower cream mixture.

10. Cover it with cheddar cheese.

11. Bake in preheated oven for 40 minutes. Serve hot.

Servings: 8

Cooking Times: 1 hour and 15 minutes

Nutrition Facts (per serving)

Calories 365

Fat 29,17g

Carbs 9,25g

Fiber 0,95g

Protein 17,9g

Baked Manchego Chicken Wings

Ingredients

20 frozen wings

1 cup of grated Manchego cheese (or Parmesan, Asagio...)

2 Tbsp. Olive oil

2 tsp. dried oregano

1/2 Tbsp. garlic powder

1 tsp. garlic salt

Directions

1. Preheat oven to 450F.

2. In a baking pan greased with olive oil place frozen chicken wings. Sprinkle with salt and oregano.

3. Bake for 35 minutes.

4. Remove from oven and toss in a bowl with another tbsp. of garlic oil until coated.

5. Sprinkle with grated Manchego cheese and garlic powder.

6. Serve hot.

Servings: 4

Cooking Times

Total Time: 45 minutes

Nutrition Facts (per serving)

Calories 446

Fat 33,51g

Carbs 2,67g

Fiber 0,68g

Protein 32,34g

Baked Pork Chops in Sweet-Sour Marinade

Ingredients

4.48 lbs. pork chops

1 cup Apple cider vinegar

1 cup Erythritol

4 Tbsp. soy Sauce

1 cup Apple Cider Vinegar

1 tsp. ginger

1 tsp. pepper

coconut or olive oil for greasing

Directions

1. Preheat oven to 350F.

2. In a food processor, add all of the ingredients (except the pork chops).

3. Blend well to make the marinade.

4. In a greased pan place all of the pork chops and pour the marinade over it.

5. Cook for 60 minutes in a preheated oven flipping after 30 minutes.

6. Once ready place chops on a serving plate and enjoy your lunch!

Servings: 10

Cooking Times

Preparation Time: 10 minutes

Total Time: 1 hour and 10 minutes

Nutrition Facts (per serving)

Calories 307

Fat 6,97g

Carbs 11,43g

Fiber 0,08g

Protein 45,89g

Bolognese Squash Spaghetti

Ingredients

1 lb. ground beef

2 1/2 cups Spaghetti squash

1 egg

3/4 cup Marinara Sauce

1 cup grated Parmesan cheese

1 cups shredded mozzarella cheese

1 tsp. chili powder

1/2 tsp. oregano

1/2 tsp. parsley (fresh and chopped)

1/2 tsp. basil

1 tsp. crushed red pepper flakes

2 tsp. of garlic minced

sea salt and ground fresh pepper to taste

ghee

Directions

1. Preheat oven to 350F.

2. Roast your spaghetti squash in the oven for about one hour.

3. In a saucepan, heat Marinara sauce; add oregano, parsley, basil and red pepper flakes. Cover and let simmer for a few minutes. Mix meatball ingredients in a bowl and roll into quarter-sized mini meatballs.

4. In a frying pan heat the ghee and cook meatballs covered. After 3 minutes, flip when halfway browned.

5. Once the meatballs are cooked through, transfer them into the sauce.

6. In a small bread pan, layer spaghetti squash, sauce, meatballs and mozzarella.

7. Bake on 25 for 30 minutes. Serve hot.

Servings: 5

Cooking Times

Total Time: 45 minutes

Nutrition Facts (per serving)

Calories 446

Fat 30,63g

Carbs 9,1g

Fiber 0,93g

Protein 32,33g

Cheesy Zoodles with Fresh Basil

Ingredients

2 cups zucchini noodles (zoodles)

2 Tbsp. fresh chopped basil

1/4 cup Pecorino Romano cheese, shaved

1/4 cup Grana Padano cheese, grated

3 Tbsp. salted butter

3 cloves mashed garlic

1 tsp. red pepper flakes

1 Tbsp. chopped red pepper

1 Tbsp. coconut oil

Salt and fresh cracked pepper to taste

Directions

1. In a frying pan over medium heat, melt butter and coconut oil. Add in garlic, chopped red pepper and red pepper flakes. Sauté for 1 minute only.

2. Add in the zoodles and let cook for 1-2 minutes. Turn off heat and toss with fresh basil. Toss slightly.

3. Add in Pecorino Romano cheese and toss.

4. Finally, sprinkle on top with grated Grana Padano cheese.

5. Serve immediately.

Servings: 3

Cooking Times

Total Time: 15 minutes

Nutrition Facts (per serving)

Calories 314

Fat 26,38g

Carbs 6,18g

Fiber 2,3g

Protein 15,78g

Spicy Spinach Casserole

Ingredients

2 1/2 cups spinach, drained

2 lbs. ground pork/beef

16 oz. cream cheese

10 Tbsp. sour cream

8 oz. Emmenthal Cheese, shredded

2 cups pepper sauce

1 onion

1 red pepper

4 tsp. Taco seasoning

Sliced Jalapeños to taste

Directions

1. Preheat oven to 350F. Grease one 8" square and a 9x13 baking dish.

2. Chop and sauté some jalapenos with chopped peppers and onions. Transfer to a bowl and set aside.

3. Add the spinach to the pan and cook until thawed completely. Move the spinach to the prep bowl

4. In a frying pan, add ground pork/meat and cook until browned well. Add taco seasoning and mix. Remove from fire and set aside.

5. In a bowl, add sour cream, mozzarella and cream cheese. Add in peppers, onion, spinach and ground meat.

6. Transfer this mix to prepared and greased baking dish and bake for 40 minutes.

7. Serve hot or cold.

Servings: 10

Cooking Times

Preparation Time: 15 minutes

Cooking Time: 45 minutes

Total Time: 1 hour

Nutrition Facts (per serving)

Calories 460

Fat 37,26g

Carbs 5,33g

Fiber 0,84g

Protein 25,63g

Cabbage with Ground Beef Stew

Ingredients

1 1/2 lb. ground beef

2 lbs. green cabbage

1/2 cup unsalted butter

1/2 cup water

3 cups pasta sauce

Salt and pepper to taste

Directions

1. In a food processor, shred quartered cabbage.

2. In a saucepan, melt the butter and add the cabbage, water and salt and pepper to taste.

3. Cover and cook for 12-15 minutes, stirring occasionally

4. In a meanwhile, in a frying pan brown the ground beefs.

5. Once browned, add the beef to the cabbage and stir well. Finally, add the pasta sauce and stir. Serve hot.

Servings: 10

Cooking Times

Cooking Time: 15 minutes

Total Time: 25 minutes

Nutrition Facts (per serving)

270

Calories 307

Total Fat 22,29g

Total Carbs 12,34g

Fiber 3,6g

Protein 14,9g

Three Cheeses & Beef Pizza

Ingredients

1 lb. ground beef

2 beef sausage

1 cup chopped Romaine lettuce

2 Tbsp. yellow onions

3 Tbsp. chopped dill pickle

1 1/2 cups Parmesan cheese

1/2 cup Colby cheese, shredded

1 1/2 cups Cheddar, shredded

1/4 Tbsp. paprika

1/4 tsp. Old Bay seasoning

1/4 tsp. garlic powder

1/4 tsp. onion powder

2 Tbsp. organic Thousand island dressing

mustard to taste

1/4 tsp. sea salt

1/4 tsp. ground black pepper

olive oil

2 Tbsp. water

Directions

1. In a frying pan greased with olive oil, add 1 cup Parmesan cheese evenly and then on top, 1 cup shredded Cheddar.

2. Leave to cook 2-3 minutes; use a spatula to lift the edges and underneath of the pizza, and slide out onto a flat surface. Allow to cool.

3. Repeat the same process, for the second pizza crust. Once done, set both cheese crusts aside.

4. Use a spatula and evenly spread Thousand Island dressing over the cheese crusts

5. In a frying pan add ground beef and cook until browned. Add old bay seasoning, garlic powder, onion powder paprika, 2 tbsp. water, salt, ground black pepper to taste. Mix and set to simmer on low.

6. Finally, add in chopped hot dogs into slices and simmer for about 4-5 minutes.

7. Place chopped lettuce over your pizza crust.

8. In a bowl, place your pickles, onions, Colby cheese, and set aside.

9. On top of each cheese crust, add about a cup of the ground meat and hotdog mixture and spread evenly .Sprinkle with onions and pickles.

10. Drizzle mustard on top.

11. Sprinkle with more cheese if you like and serve.

Servings: 7

Cooking Time: 20 minutes

Nutrition Facts (per serving)

Calories 511

Fat 39,9g

Carbs 2,78g

Fiber 0,42g

Protein 33,59g

Chicken Angel Eggs

Ingredients

1 cup chicken, finely chopped

6 eggs

3 Tbsp. mayonnaise

1 Tbsp. chopped onion

1/2 tsp. dill

1/2 tsp. parsley

1 tsp. Dijon mustard

1/2 tsp. pepper mix seasoning

old bay seasoning

salt and black ground pepper to taste

Directions

1. In a bowl, mix all rest of ingredients (except eggs) until well mixed. Refrigerate the chicken salad for 10-15 minutes.

2. Boil your eggs. Shell, cool, and cut in half. Save or toss your yolks.

3. Fill your egg halves with chicken salad. Sprinkle with Old Bay or some other seasoning of your taste. Serve.

Servings: 4

Cooking Times

Total Time: 25 minutes

Nutrition Facts (per serving)

Calories 161

Fat 11,22g

Carbs 3,73g

Fiber 0,08g

Protein 10,82g

Monterey Jack Steak

Ingredients

1 lb. shaved steak

4 slices Monterey Jack cheese

2 Tbsp. mayonnaise

1 Tbsp. Dijon mustard

1/4 cup chopped green peppers

1/4 cup chopped onions

1 Tbsp. minced garlic

1 Tbsp. olive oil

1 Tbsp. ghee

Directions

1. In a large frying pan add ghee and olive oil to warm over medium heat. Add onions, green peppers and garlic. Cook until soft, about 2-3 minutes. Add shaved steak and cook until browned several minutes.

2. Turn heat down to low. Add Dijon mustard and mayonnaise and mix.

3. Add Monterey Jack cheese on top of the steak and let melt until cheese is melted throughout, about 1 minute.

4. Serve hot.

Servings: 4

Cooking Times

Total Time: 20 minutes

Nutrition Facts (per serving)

Calories 345

Fat 25,2g

Carbs 4,35g

Fiber 0,48g

Protein 24,51g

Pumpkin Chili

Ingredients

2 lbs. ground beef

1 can (15 oz.) pumpkin puree

1 Tbsp. pumpkin pie spice

3 cups 100% tomato juice

3 tomatoes, diced

1 red bell pepper

1 yellow onion

2 tsp. cumin

1 Tbsp. chili powder

2 tsp. cayenne pepper

ghee or coconut oil

Directions

1. In a large frying pan greased with ghee or coconut oil, brown the meat over medium heat.

2. Chop the onion and pepper and add into the pot with the meat. Cook 3-5 minutes or until the onions become translucent.

3. Add in the rest of the ingredients and let simmer on LOW for 30 minutes.

4. Season chili with salt and pepper to taste and cook for another 30 minutes.

5. Serve hot.

Servings: 8

Cooking Times

Total Time: 1 hour and 20 minutes

Nutrition Facts (per serving)

Calories 354

Fat 25,24g

Carbs 9,87g

Fiber 2,14g 9%

Protein 21,87g 44%

Slow Cooker Roast and Chicken Stew

Ingredients

3 lb. pot roast

1 lb. chicken breast (boiled and shredded)

6 oz. Italian sweet sausage

2 cups beef broth

1 cup chicken stock

1/2 medium onion (chopped)

1 can (11 oz.) low carb diced tomatoes

1/4 tsp. thyme

1/4 tsp. celery salt

1 Tbsp. coconut oil

1 tsp. basil

2 tsp. dried dill weed

2 tsp. garlic powder

2 tsp. pepper

1 Tbsp. garlic salt

1 tsp. minced garlic

1 Tbsp. oregano

1 Tbsp. powdered buttermilk

4 tsp. onion powder

4 tsp. dried parsley

5 tsp. red pepper flakes

2 tsp. hot sauce

Directions

1. At the bottom of your Slow Cooker place roast, chicken breast and Italian sausages. Add on the top all other ingredients and stir lightly.
2. Close the lid and cook on LOW for about 6-8 hours.
3. Once ready, flavor to taste with some additional hot sauce, salt and pepper to your own liking and serve hot.

Servings: 10

Nutrition Facts (per serving)
Calories 467
Fat 36,21g
Carbs 3,76g
Fiber 1,03g
Protein 30,11g

Mediterranean Pecorino Romano Breaded Cutlets

Ingredients

6 pork cutlets

1/2 cup grated Pecorino Romano cheese

2 Tbsp. fresh lemon juice

2 Tbsp. water

1 Tbsp. olive oil

1 Tbsp. green pepper, minced

1 Tbsp. garlic, minced

salt and ground black pepper to taste

Directions

1. Heat a greasing frying pan to medium.
2. In a bowl pour water, lemon juice, olive oil, minced pepper and garlic. Season the salt and pepper to taste. Mix well.
3. In a separate bowl pour grated Pecorino Romano cheese.
4. Dip each cutlet first in liquid dressing and then in cheese.
5. Cook cutlets in pan for about 15-20 minutes. Serve hot.

Servings: 3

Cooking Times

Total Time: 30 minutes

Nutrition Facts (per serving)

Calories 395

Fat 38,78g

Carbs 2,5g

Fiber 0,16g

Protein 9,1g

Oriental Garlicky Chicken Thighs

Ingredients

4 chicken thighs

16 whole cloves of garlic

2 Tbsp. ghee

2 Tbsp. juice of one fresh lemon

1 cup of baby carrots

1 onion, cut into quarters

2 tomatoes cut in half

3 Tbsp. garlic olive oil (or extra-virgin olive oil)

oregano

Salt and pepper

Directions

1. Preheat oven to 500F degrees.
2. Grease the bottom of a non-stick frying pan with garlic olive oil (or olive oil). Add in the chicken thighs together.
3. In between the thighs, wedge in the garlic gloves, onions, tomatoes and baby carrots.
4. Pour the lemon juice over the chicken thighs. Drizzle ghee and garlic oil over the thighs.
5. Sprinkle oregano over the dish and season with salt and pepper to taste.
6. Bake in preheated oven for 25-30 minutes.
7. Reduce heat to 350 and cook for 20 minutes more.
8. Once ready, let cool for 5 minutes on a wire rack and serve hot.

Servings: 4

Cooking Times

Total Time: 1 hour and 5 minutes

Nutrition Facts (per serving)

Calories 237

Fat 14,52g

Carbs 8,97g

Fiber 1,31g

Protein 17,68g

Pordenone Cauliflower Lasagna

Ingredients

12 chicken thighs

30 oz. chopped cauliflower

6 green onions

1 onion, chopped

1 green pepper

6 bacon Slices

1 cup Cream Cheese

1/2 cup heavy cream

8 oz. Pepper Jack Cheese, shredded

8 oz. Cheddar Cheese, shredded

1 Tbsp. garlic, minced

salt and pepper to taste

Directions

1. Preheat oven to350F.
2. Chop up a head of cauliflower into florets. Cook the cauliflower in the microwave on the vegetable setting. Set aside.
3. In a pan on stovetop, toss the chicken thighs with salt and pepper to taste. Add some water to about mid-thigh and cook for 60 minutes. Chop up the onions and peppers and pan fry it.
4. Add all of the other ingredients, reserving 2 oz. Cheddar and 2 oz. of Pepper Jack Cheese.
5. Add the mixture into a large, greased casserole dish and top with the remaining cheese.
6. Cover with foil and cook for 30 minutes. Serve hot.

Servings: 10

Cooking Times

Preparation Time: 20 minutes

Cooking Time: 1 hour and 30 minutes

Nutrition Facts (per serving)

Calories 486

Fat 35,69g

Carbs 13,73g

Fiber 2,2g

Protein 28,09g

Roasted Chicken & Prosciutto with Brussels sprouts

Ingredients

2 lbs. chicken tenderloins

4 oz. prosciutto

12 oz. Brussels sprouts

1/2 cup chicken broth

1 1/2 cups heavy cream

1 tsp. minced garlic

1 lemon, quartered and seeded

ghee or coconut oil for frying

Directions

1. Preheat oven to 400 degrees.

2. Cut the Brussels sprouts in half and boil for 5 minutes. Remove from heat and set aside.

3. In a frying pan add 1/2 cup chicken broth and bring to a boil on medium. After that, add heavy cream, minced garlic and lemon and let simmer for 5-10 minutes stirring frequently. Remove from heat and set aside.

4. In a separate frying pan, heat up some ghee and add chicken. Cook on medium high heat for several minutes, and then add chopped prosciutto until chicken is cooked.

5. In a small casserole dish (9×9) and layer from bottom to top: Brussels sprouts, chicken, prosciutto, lemon cream sauce on top.

6. Bake in preheated oven for 20 minutes. Serve hot.

Servings: 6

Cooking Times

Total Time: 40 minutes

Nutrition Facts (per serving)

Calories 333

Fat 16,76g

Carbs 5,2g

Fiber 1,48g

Protein 39,47g

Roquefort Spinach, Zoodles and Bacon Salad

Ingredients

4 cups of zucchini noodles

1 cup fresh broccoli

1/2 cup crumbled bacon

1 cup fresh spinach

1/3 cup Roquefort, bleu cheese, crumbled

1/3 cup bleu cheese dressing

fresh cracked pepper (to taste)

Directions

1. In a deep bowl add all the ingredients together and toss slightly with wooden spoon.
2. Serve and enjoy!

Servings: 5

Cooking Time: 5 minutes

Nutrition Facts (per serving)

Calories 81,

Fat 3,15g

Carbs 9,58g

Fiber 3,05g

Protein 6,07g

Sour Avocado and Chicken Moussaka

Ingredients

8 chicken thighs, cooked

1 cup sour cream

1 cup Parmesan Cheese

4 avocados

1 onion

1 green pepper

1 Tbsp. cayenne peppers sauce

salt and ground pepper to taste

coconut oil for greasing

Directions

1. Preheat oven to 350 F. Grease a baking dish with coconut oil.

2. In a pot cook your chicken thighs about 35 minutes. Peel avocados, cut in half, and slice into thin strips.

3. Line the bottom with avocado slices. In a small pan fry chopped peppers and onions until caramelized.

4. Add the chicken into a large bowl and chop it. Add remaining ingredients and mix well.

5. Spoon mixture over the avocado slices. Bake for 20 minutes.

6. Serve hot.

Servings: 8

Cooking Times

Total Time: 35 minutes

Nutrition Facts (per serving)

Calories 345

Fat 25,32g

Carbs 11,08g

Fiber 6,45g

Protein 20,98g

Spicy Italian Sausage and Spinach Casserole

Ingredients

16 oz. spicy Italian sausage

2 1/2 cups frozen spinach

12 eggs

8 oz. Cheddar

1 onion

9 oz. Cherry Tomatoes

1 green pepper, chopped

12 Tbsp. Heavy Cream

Garlic powder

Onion Powder

Salt and ground pepper to taste

coconut or olive oil

Directions

1. Preheat oven to 350F. Grease casserole dish with coconut or olive oil.

2. In microwave cook the spinach. Chop the spicy Italian sausage and cook in a frying pan until browned. Remove to the big bowl and set aside.

3. In the same frying pan, cook the sliced onion and pepper. Transfer to the bowl with spinach.

4. Whisk together the eggs, spices and a heavy cream. Add the cheese to the bowl and combine, then add the egg mixture and combine.

5. Transfer to a greased casserole dish and add cherry tomatoes.

6. Cook in preheated oven for 50 minutes. Serve hot.

Servings: 10

Cooking Times

Total Time: 1 hour and 5 minutes

Nutrition Facts (per serving)

Calories 343

Fat 25,91g

Carbs 6,27g

Fiber 2,5g

Protein 22,68g

Squash Spaghetti Lasagna Dish

Ingredients

2 1/2 lbs. ground beef

2 large Spaghetti Squash

7 ounces whole milk Ricotta Cheese

7 ounces Mozzarella cheese, sliced

4 cups Marinara sauce

coconut or olive oil for greasing

Directions

1. Preheat oven to 375F. Grease a large baking dish with coconut or olive oil.

2. Split the Spaghetti Squash and lay face down into large glass dish and fill with water. Bake for 40-45 minutes.

3. While the Spaghetti Squash is cooking, in a large saucepan cook the ground meat and the marinara sauce. Once combined, set aside.

4. When the Spaghetti Squash is done scrap the meat of the squash to from spaghetti.

5. Assembly the lasagna in a large greased pan, start with a layer of Spaghetti Squash, then the meat sauce, then slices of mozzarella, then ricotta, then repeats until ingredients are exhausted.

6. Bake for 30-35 35 minutes until the top layer of cheese is browning. Serve hot or keep refrigerated.

Servings: 14

Cooking Times

Total Time: 1 hour and 30 minutes

Nutrition Facts (per serving)

Calories 437,

Fat 27,77g

Carbs 16,49g

Fiber 1,91g

Protein 28,79g

Tuna Avocado Bites

Ingredients

Mayonnaise (1/4 cup)

Parmesan cheese (1/4 cup)

Garlic powder (1/2 teaspoon)

Salt

Canned Tuna (10 oz., drained)

Avocado (1, cubed)

Almond flour (1/3 cup)

Onion powder (1/4 teaspoon)

Coconut oil (1/2 cup)

Directions

1. Combine all ingredients in a bowl except oil and avocado.
2. Add avocado and fold, use hands to form balls and dust with flour.
3. Heat oil in a pot and fry tuna bites until golden all over.
4. Serve.

Servings: 12

Nutrition Facts (per serving)

Calories 135

Fats 11.8g

Protein 6.2 g

298

Fiber 1.2g

Note: 3-4 bites would be good for a serving. Paired with a salad and lunch is complete.

Crispy Baked Tofu and Bok Choy Salad

Ingredients

For Tofu:

Soy sauce (1 tablespoon)

Water (1 tablespoon)

Rice wine vinegar (1 tablespoon)

Tofu (15 oz., extra firm)

Sesame oil (1 tablespoon)

Garlic (2 teaspoons)

Lemon juice (from ½ lemon)

For Salad:

Green onion (1 stalk)

Coconut oil (3 tablespoons)

Sambal Olek (1 tablespoon)

Lime juice (from ½ lime)

Bok Choy (9 oz.)

Cilantro (2 tablespoons, chopped)

Soy sauce (2 tablespoons)

Peanut butter (1 tablespoon)

Stevia liquid (7 drops)

Directions
1. Wrap tofu in a clean cloth and press for 6 hours until dry.
2. Combine soy sauce, water, vinegar, lemon juice, sesame oil and garlic in a bowl and cube tofu. Add to marinade, cover with plastic and put aside for 30 minutes or overnight if possible.
3. Set oven to 350 ℉. Use parchment paper to line a baking sheet and place marinated tofu on sheet. Bake for 35 minutes.

4. Prepare dressing for salad by combining all ingredients except bok choy. Chop bok choy finely and toss in dressing.
5. Top bok choy with baked tofu and serve.

Servings: 3

Nutrition Facts (per serving)
Calories 442
Net Carbs 5.7g
Fats 35g
Protein 25 g
Fiber 1.7g

Homemade Meatballs

Ingredients

500g ground beef

1 whole egg

Almond flour (1/2 cups)

2 cloves of garlic, minced

Oregano, dried (1 teaspoon)

Thyme, dried (1 teaspoon)

1 cup mozzarella cheese, shredded

Salt and pepper to taste

Homemade marinara sauce (1/2 cups)

Directions

1. Preheat oven at 450F.

2. In a large bowl, place the ground beef, egg, almond flour, garlic, oregano, thyme, and season with salt and pepper. Also add the cheese.

3. Using your hands, mix all the ingredients together; making sure that everything is well combined.

4. Create 25 pcs of meat balls and lay them on a baking sheet lined with parchment paper.

5. Cook in the oven to cook for 15 minutes or until golden brown.

6. Serve the meatballs with marinara sauce.

Servings: 12

Nutrition Facts (per serving)

Calories: 117

Net Carbs: 0.9

Fat: 9.3g

Protein: 7g

BBQ Chicken Soup

Ingredients

For Soup Base:

Chicken thighs (3)

Salt

Chicken broth (1 ½ cups)

Chili seasoning (2 teaspoons)

Olive oil (2 tablespoons)

Beef broth (1 ½ cups)

Black pepper

For BBQ Sauce:

Ketchup (1/4 cup, reduced sugar)

Dijon mustard (2 tablespoons)

Hot sauce (1 tablespoon)

Worcestershire sauce (1 teaspoon)

Onion powder (1 teaspoon)

Red chili flakes (1 teaspoon)

Butter (1/4 cup)

Tomato paste (1/4 cup)

Soy sauce (1 tablespoon)

Liquid smoke (2 ½ teaspoons)

Garlic powder (1 ½ teaspoons)

Chili powder (1 teaspoon)

Cumin (1 teaspoon)

Directions

1. Set oven to 400°F. Remove bones from chicken and put bones aside. Season chicken with chili seasoning and place into oven for 50 minutes.

2. Heat oil in a deep pot and add bones. Cook for 5 minutes then add beef and chicken broth; season with pepper and salt.

3. Take chicken from oven and remove skin. Add the fat to the soup and mix together. Combine BBQ sauce ingredients and add to pot. Cook for 30 minutes.

4. Combine fats in soup by using an immersion blender then shred chicken and add to soup. Cook for 20 minutes.

5. Serve topped with chicken skin. May add cheese or bell peppers.

Servings: 4

Nutrition Facts (per serving)

Calories 487

Net Carbs 4.3g

Fats 38.3g

Protein 24.5 g

Fiber 1.3g

Salmon Salad in Avo Cups

Ingredients

1 medium-sized salmon fillet

1 pc. shallot, diced

Mayo (1/4 cups)

½ juice of lime

Fresh dill, chopped (2 tablespoons)

Ghee (1 tablespoon)

1 large avocado, sliced in half and pitted

salt and pepper to taste

Directions

1. Preheat oven at 400F

2. Place the salmon fillet on a baking sheet and drizzle it with ghee and juice of lime. Season with salt and pepper and place in the oven to cook for 20-25 minutes.

3. When done, allow the salmon to cook for a few minutes and shred using a fork.

4. Place the salmon in a bowl, add the diced shallot, and mix well.

5. Add the dill and mayo to the salmon mixture and combine well. Set aside.

6. Remove the insides of the avocado halves making sure that the skin is still intact to make cups.

7. Mash the avocado meat in a bowl and then add to the salmon mixture. Combine well.

8. Transfer the avocado and salmon salad back to the avocado cups and serve.

Servings: 2

Nutrition Facts (per serving)

Calories: 463

Net Carbs: 6.4g

Fat: 35g

Protein: 27g

Bacon Chicken Patties

Ingredients

Chicken breast (12 oz. can)

Bell peppers (2, medium)

Parmesan cheese (1/4 cup)

Coconut flour (3 tablespoons)

Bacon (4 slices)

Sundried Tomato pesto (1/4 cup)

Egg (1)

Directions

1. Cook bacon until crisp, put aside until needed.

2. Put bell pepper into a processor and pulse until fine, put into a bowl and squeeze out excess liquid.

3. Put bacon and chicken into processor and pulse until thoroughly combined, transfer mixture to bowl with peppers.

4. Add egg, pesto parmesan and flour to mixture and combine.

5. Heat oil in a skillet and form patties. Add to pan and cook until golden all over.

6. Serve.

Servings: 10

Nutrition Facts (per serving)

Calories 159

Net Carbs 1.7g

Fats 11.5g

Protein 9.9 g

Fiber 14g

Savory Mince

Ingredients

Coconut oil (4 tablespoons)

1Kg Beef/Chicken/Lamb/Pork/Ostrich mince

2 Onion finely diced

Vegetables (green/red/yellow/orange peppers, mushroom, tomatoes, celery, baby marrows, spinach) finely diced (4 cups)

4 Carrots finely grated

1 Packet gluten free gravy

Tomato paste (1/2 cups)

250ml chicken stock

Directions

1. Heat coconut oil in a pan and fry chopped onion,

2. Add beef mince with and tomato paste and fry.

3. Add chopped vegetables and grated carrot to the cooked mince.

4. Continue to cook on a low heat until the vegetables are well cooked.

5. If your mixture seems to be drying out, keep adding chicken stock to keep at the right consistency.

6. The longer you cook this mixture, the more the flavours will infuse through the mince.

7. Add gluten free gravy

Cheesy Bacon Spinach Log

Ingredients

Cheddar cheese (2 ½ cups, shredded)

Chipotle seasoning (2 tablespoons)

Bacon (30 slices)

Mrs. Dash seasoning (2 teaspoons)

Spinach (5 cups)

Directions

1. Set oven to 375 F.

2. Place bacon in a weaving pattern on a baking sheet lined with foil and season with spices.

3. Top bacon with cheese leaving a 1 inch space all around the edge. Add spinach and push it down and roll the bacon together into a log.

4. Sprinkle with salt and place into oven for 60 minutes.

5. Cool for 15 minutes and slice.

6. Serve.

Servings: 5

Nutrition Facts (per serving)

Calories 432

Net Carbs 3g

Fats 38.2g

Protein 32.8 g

Fiber 3g

Beef Sausage, Bacon & Broccoli Casserole

Ingredients

500 g beef sausage

1/2 head of broccoli

8 slices of bacon

Cream (1/2 cups)

Dijon mustard (1 tablespoon)

100 g grated cheddar cheese

Directions

1. Preheat oven to 350F

2. Slice the sausage and place in a small baking dish.

3. Slice the bacon and add to the sausage.

4. Break the broccoli into florets and arrange between the meat.

5. Mix the cream and mustard in a bowl and pour it all over the casserole, then top with the cheese.

6. Bake in the oven for 35 minutes.

Servings: 2

Nutrition Facts (per serving)

Calories: 300

Net Carbs: 3g

Fat: 25g

Protein: 20g

Grilled Cheese and Ham Sandwich

Ingredients

For buns:

Eggs (2)

Salted butter (1 ½ tablespoons)

Coconut flour (1 teaspoon)

Almond flour (3/4 cup)

Coconut oil (2 tablespoons)

Baking powder (1 teaspoon)

Salt (1/4 teaspoon)

Filling:

Deli Ham (4 slices)

Cheddar cheese (2 slices)

Butter (1 tablespoon, salted)

Muenster cheese (2 slices)

Directions

1. Set oven to 350 F.

2. Place almond flour, baking powder in a bowl and mix together.

3. Put coconut oil and butter in a microwavable dish and heat until melted then add to dry mix. Combine until mixture gets doughy.

4. Beat eggs and add to dough mixture then put in coconut flour.

5. Grease cupcake molds and add batter to each about ¾ ways filled. Baked for 18 minutes and take from oven, allow to cool and slice into two horizontally.

6. Use cheese and ham to fill buns, melt butter in a skillet and place sandwiches into pan. Cook for 3 minutes on each side until golden and cheese melts.

7. Serve.

Servings: 1

Nutrition Facts (per serving)

Calories 272

Fats 24.2g

Protein 11.3g

Fiber 3.8g

Creamed Spinach

Ingredients

Spinach (2 cups)

½ small onion, chopped

Water (1/4 cups)

1/2 stock cube

1 clove of garlic, chopped

Heavy cream (1/4 cups)

Butter (2 tablespoons)

Salt and pepper to taste

Directions

1. Place spinach and onion to a pan with water and heat over medium-high fire.

2. Add stock cube and garlic and allow to steam for 8-10 minutes or until all the water has evaporated and the spinach is very soft.

3. Pour in the heavy cream and butter and then season with salt and pepper. Cooking until it thickens.

4. Using a hand-held blender blitz the spinach until fairly smooth.

5. Serve while hot

Servings: 1

Nutrition Facts (per serving)

Calories: 200

Net Carbs: 3g

Fat: 23g

Protein: 7g

Cheesy Pizza

Ingredients

Ground beef (1/2 lb.)

Eggs (2)

Garlic powder (1 teaspoon)

Basil (1/4 teaspoon)

Turmeric (1/4 teaspoon)

Cream cheese (8 oz., room temp.)

Chorizo sausage (1)

Parmesan cheese (1/4 cup, grated)

Cumin (1/2 teaspoon)

Italian seasoning (1/2 teaspoon)

Tomato sauce (3/4 cup, low carb)

Salt

Black pepper

Directions

1. Set oven to 375 F.
2. Put cream cheese, eggs, garlic powder, parmesan cheese and black pepper in a bowl and use mixer to blend until smooth.
3. Grease a baking pan and pour in cheese mixture and spread evenly; bake for 15 minutes.
4. Put beef into a skillet and cook for 5 minutes then add Italian seasoning, basil, salt, black pepper, cumin and turmeric. Cook for 10 minutes or until thoroughly cooked.
5. Take crust from oven and cool for 10 minutes then top with tomato sauce and cheese. Return to oven and bake for 10 minutes until cheese melts then top with beef.

6. Broil for an additional 5 minutes. Take from oven and cool for 10 minutes.

7. Slice and serve.

Servings: 12 small slices

Nutrition Facts (per serving)

Calories 145

Net Carbs 1.2g

Fats 11.3g

Protein 8.2 g

Fiber 3g

Hearty Portobello Burgers

Ingredients

Coconut oil (1/2 tablespoon)

Oregano (1 teaspoon)

Portobello mushroom caps (2)

Garlic (1 clove)

Salt

Black pepper

Dijon mustard (1 tablespoon)

Cheddar cheese (1/4 cup)

Beef/bison (6 oz.)

Directions

1. Heat griddle and combine spices and oil in a bowl.

2. Remove gills from mushrooms and place into marinade until needed.

3. Add beef, cheese, salt, mustard and pepper in another bowl and mix to combine; form into a patty.

4. Place marinated caps onto grill and cook for 8 minutes until thoroughly heated. Place patty onto grill and cook on each side for 5 minutes.

5. Take 'buns' from grill and top with burger and any other toppings you choose.

6. Serve.

Servings: 1

Nutrition Facts (per serving)

Calories 735

Net Carbs 4g

Fats 48g

Protein 60g

Fiber 4g

Chicken and Broccoli filled Zucchini

Ingredients

Butter (2 tablespoons)

Broccoli (1 cup)

Sour cream (2 tablespoons)

Zucchini (10 oz.)-2

Cheddar cheese (3 oz., shredded)

Rotisserie chicken (6 oz., shredded)

Green onion (1 stalk)

Salt

Black pepper

Directions

1. Set oven to 400 F.

2. Slice zucchinis in half lengthwise and use spoons to remove cores. Melt butter and pour equally into each zucchini shell. Add black pepper and salt and bake for 20 minutes.

3. Chop broccoli and place into a bowl with sour cream and chicken. Fill zucchini boats with chicken mixture and top with cheese.

4. Bake for 15 minutes more or until golden.

5. Serve topped with green onion.

Servings: 2

Nutrition Facts (per serving)

Calories 476.5

Net Carbs 5g

Fats 34g

Protein 30 g

Fiber 3g

Super-Fast Egg Drop Soup

Ingredients

Chicken broth (1 ½ cups)

Butter (1 tablespoon)

Chili garlic paste (1 teaspoon)

Chicken bouillon (1/2 cube)

Eggs (2)

Directions

1. Add butter to pan, heat until it melts then add broth and bouillon

2. Bring to a boil and add chili paste, stir to combine and remove from flame.

3. Beat eggs in a bowl and add to broth, stir and put aside for a few minutes.

4. Serve.

Servings: 2

Nutrition Facts (per serving)

Calories 279

Net Carbs 2.5g

Fats 23g

Protein 12g

Salmon Salad in Avocado Cups

Ingredients

1 medium-sized salmon fillet

1 pc. Shallot, diced

¼ cup mayo

½ juice of lime

2 tsps. Fresh dill, chopped

1 tbsp. ghee

1 large avocado, sliced in half and pitted

salt and pepper to taste

Directions

1. Preheat oven at 400F

2. Place the salmon fillet on a baking sheet and drizzle it with ghee and juice of lime. Season with salt and pepper and place in the oven to cook for 20-25 minutes.

3. When done, allow the salmon to cook for a few minutes and shred using a fork.

4. Place the salmon in a bowl, add the diced shallot, and mix well.

5. Add the dill and mayo to the salmon mixture and combine well. Set aside.

6. Remove the insides of the avocado halves making sure that the skin is still intact to make cups.

7. Mash the avocado meat in a bowl and then add to the salmon mixture. Combine well.

8. Transfer the avocado and tuna salad back to the avocado cups and serve.

Servings: 2

Nutrition Facts (per serving)

Calories: 463

Net Carbs: 6.4g

Fat: 35g

Protein: 27g

Cheesy Hotdog Pockets

Ingredients

2 pcs. beef hot dogs

2 thick sticks of quick-melt cheese (or mozzarella)

4 slices of bacon

1/8 tsp. garlic powder

1/8 tsp. onion powder

salt and pepper to taste

Directions

1. Preheat oven at 400F

2. Cut the hotdogs lengthwise to create slits.

3. Insert the cheese sticks in the hotdog and then wrap the bacon with to the beef hotdog. Secure the bacon using a toothpick.

4. Transfer the hotdogs on a baking sheet lined with foil and flavor with garlic and onion powder.

5. Place in the oven to cook for 40 minutes or until the hotdogs turns golden brown and the cheese is melted,

6. Serve with a veggie salad on the side.

Nutritional Info (per serving)

Calories: 378

Net Carbs: 0.3 g

Fat: 35g

Protein: 17g

Beef Shred Salad

Ingredients

2 cups beef, shredded

1 yellow pepper, sliced thin lengthwise

1 white onion, sliced lengthwise

6 pcs. butter lettuce

2 tsp. mayo

1/8 tsp. chili flakes

Directions

1. Place the butter lettuces on a serving plate. Spread mayo on the lettuce and top with the shredded beef.

2. Place pepper slices and onions on top and season with chili flakes.

3. Serve as it is or rolled.

Nutritional Info (per serving)

Calories: 338

Net Carbs: 2.4

Fat: 25g

Protein: 24g

Spicy Chicken Thighs

Ingredients

2 lb. chicken thighs

¼ cup ghee or olive oil

½ tsp. garlic powder

½ tsp. paprika

½ tsp. cumin, ground

¼ tsp. cayenne

¼ tsp. coriander, ground

1/8 tsp. cinnamon, ground

1/8 tsp. ginger powder

1 tsp. salt

1 tsp. yellow curry

Directions

1. Preheat oven at 425F.

2. In a small bowl mix all the spices to create a dry rub.

3. Pat dry the chicken using a kitchen paper towel and place on a baking sheet lined with greased parchment paper.

4. Generously brush the chicken with ghee or olive oil.

5. Rub the spices to the chicken thighs making sure that you cover every side.

6. Place the chicken in the oven to cook for 50 minutes.

7. Let it cool before serving.

Nutritional Info (per serving)

Calories: 227

Net Carbs: .6g

Fat: 20g

Protein: 21g

Spring Roll in a Bowl

Ingredients

500g pork mince

2 cups cabbage, shredded finely

2 cup grated carrot

2 cups grated baby marrows

1 cup mushrooms

4 tbsp. coconut Oil

1/2 cup soya sauce

1 cup chicken stock

2 tsp. vinegar

5 cloves garlic, minced

4 tsp. grated ginger

4 finely sliced spring onions

½ cup toasted sesame seeds

1 hard-boiled egg, chopped

Directions

1.   Heat the coconut oil and fry the garlic, spring onions, ginger.

2.   Add the pork mince and brown.

3.   Add the cabbage and carrot to the pot and toss to combine. Stir in the soy sauce.

4.   Cover and cook until the vegetables are soft, about 15 minutes.

5.   Dish up; add chopped hard-boiled egg over each of the bowls.

6.   Garnish with sesame seeds once you have dished up.

Nutritional Info (per serving)

Calories: 80

Net Carbs: 5g

Fat: 5g

Protein: 3g

Green Salad

Ingredients

1 cup green beans, steamed lightly

1 cup broccoli florets, steamed lightly

1 small tomato, finely sliced

1 cup lettuce

1 round feta

¼ cup toasted sunflower seeds, roasted

1 hard-boiled egg, chopped

For dressing:

1 tbsp. olive oil

Salt and pepper to taste

Juice from ½ lemon

Directions

1. Place all the vegetables in a salad bowl.

2. Crumble the feta and sprinkle it along with the roasted pumpkin seeds and egg on top of the salad.

3. In a small bowl, pour the olive oil, add lemon juice, then add salt and pepper, and whisk together. Drizzle this dressing on top of the salad.

4. Toss gently before serving.

Nutritional Info (per serving)

Calories: 45

Net Carbs: 3g

Fat: 3g

Protein: 1g

Spinach Cheese & Bacon Log

Ingredients

Cheddar cheese (2 ½ cups, shredded)

Chipotle seasoning (2 tablespoons)

Bacon (30 slices)

Mrs. Dash seasoning (2 teaspoons)

Spinach (5 cups)

Directions

1. Set oven to 375°F.

2. Place bacon in a weaving pattern on a baking sheet lined with foil and season with spices.

3. Top bacon with cheese leaving a 1 inch space all around the edge. Add spinach and push it down and roll the bacon together into a log.

4. Sprinkle with salt and place into oven for 60 minutes.

5. Cool for 15 minutes and slice.

6. Serve.

Servings: 5

Nutrition Facts (per serving)

Calories 432

Net Carbs 3g

Fats 38.2g

Protein 32.8 g

Fiber 3g

Zucchini Stuffed with Chicken & Broccoli

Ingredients

Butter (2 tablespoons)

Broccoli (1 cup)

Sour cream (2 tablespoons)

Zucchini (10 oz.)-2

Cheddar cheese (3 oz., shredded)

Rotisserie chicken (6 oz., shredded)

Green onion (1 stalk)

Salt

Black pepper

Directions

1. Set oven to 400 °F.

2. Slice zucchinis in half lengthwise and use spoons to remove cores. Melt butter and pour equally into each zucchini shell. Add black pepper and salt and bake for 20 minutes.

3. Chop broccoli and place into a bowl with sour cream and chicken. Fill zucchini boats with chicken mixture and top with cheese.

4. Bake for 15 minutes more or until golden.

5. Serve topped with green onion.

Servings: 2

Nutrition Facts (per serving)

Calories 476.5

Net Carbs 5g

Fats 34g

Protein 30 g

Fiber 3g

Beef Pumpkin Chili

Ingredients

2 lbs. ground beef

1 can (15 oz.) pumpkin puree

1 Tbsp. pumpkin pie spice

3 cups 100% tomato juice

3 tomatoes, diced

1 red bell pepper

1 yellow onion

2 tsp. cumin

1 Tbsp. chili powder

2 tsp. cayenne pepper

ghee or coconut oil

Directions

1. In a large frying pan greased with ghee or coconut oil, brown the meat over medium heat.

2. Chop the onion and pepper and add into the pot with the meat. Cook 3-5 minutes or until the onions become translucent.

3. Add in the rest of the ingredients and let simmer on LOW for 30 minutes.

4. Season chili with salt and pepper to taste and cook for another 30 minutes.

5. Serve hot.

Servings: 8

Cooking Time: 1 hour and 20 minutes

Nutrition Facts (per serving)

Calories 354, 83

Fat 25,24g

Fiber 2,14g

Sugar 5,5g

Protein 21,87g

BLT Roll

Ingredients

4 leaves, romaine lettuce

4 bacon strips, cooked and crumbled

4 slices deli turkey

1 cup cherry tomatoes, cut in half

2 tbsp. mayonnaise

Directions

1. Lay the turkey slice on top of the lettuce leaves.
2. Spread mayonnaise on the turkey slice and then top with the cherry tomatoes and bacon on top.
3. Roll the lettuce and then secure with toothpick.
4. Serve immediately.

Serves 1

Nutritional Information

Calories 382

Net Carbs 11.5g

Fats 38.5g

Protein 4.1g

Fiber 6.3g

2-Cheese and Bacon Soup

Ingredients

3 bacon strips, cooked and chopped

1 cup cheddar, shredded

1 cup Monterey jack cheese, shredded

1 small bell pepper, chopped

2 cloves of garlic, minced

1 onion, chopped fine

12 oz. gluten-free beer

½ cup milk

½ cup light cream

2 tbsp. butter

2 tbsp. flour

salt and pepper to taste

Directions

1. Using the grease from cooking bacon, sauté the onions and bell pepper for 5 minutes in a pot over medium heat.
2. Adjust the heat to low and add the garlic and cook for another 2 minutes.
3. Increase the heat again and then add the 2 tbsp. butter and allow it to boil.
4. Add the 2 tbsp. flour to the pot and whisk for 3 minutes.
5. Pour the beer and stir constantly for 5 minutes.
6. Lower the heat again and add the milk and light cream.
7. Remove the pot from the head and then add the cheese. Stir until the cheese has completely melted.
8. Season with salt and pepper and transfer into serving bowls.

9.   Garnish with crispy bacon on top. Serve hot.

Serves 4-5

Nutritional Information

Calories 442

Net Carbs 11g

Fats 34g

Protein 20g

Cauliflower and Cheese Chowder

Ingredients

4 cups cauliflower florets, chopped

4 bacon strips

1 tbsp. organic butter

2 cloves of garlic, minced

1 onion, chopped fine

¼ almond flour

4 cups low-sodium chicken broth

½ cup milk

¼ cup light cream

1 cup cheddar, shredded

salt and pepper to taste

Directions

1. Cook the bacon in a large pot. Remove from the pot when cooked and set aside.

2. Using the same pot, set the heat on medium and throw in the onions. Cook for 3 minutes and then add the garlic and cauliflower florets and cook for another 5 minutes.

3. Add the flour into the pot and continuously whisk for a minute.

4. Pour the chicken broth, milk, and light cream and stir for 3 minutes.

5. Allow to simmer for 15 minutes and then turn off the heat.

6. Add the cheddar cheese into the pot, season with salt and pepper and stir again.

7. Serve with the chopped bacon on top.

Serves 4

Nutritional Information

Calories 268

Net Carbs 11.9g

Fats 15.9g

Protein 19.5g

Fiber 3.1g

Pizza in Mushroom Cups

Ingredients

3 large Portobello mushroom caps

3 tsp. pizza seasoning

3 tomato, slices

½ cup fresh basil leaves, chopped

12 slices pepperoni

¼ cup mozzarella cheese

¼ cup cheddar cheese

¼ cup Monterey jack

½ tbsp. olive oil

Directions

1. Set the oven at 450F
2. Place the mushroom caps on a baking sheet lined with parchment paper and drizzle with olive oil
3. Season with the pizza seasoning and top with the basil, tomato slices, cheeses, and season again.
4. Place in the oven to bake for 5-6 minutes or until the cheese has melted
5. Get the baking sheet out of the oven and then top with the pepperoni and place back in the oven and bake until the pepperoni is cooked.

Makes 3

Nutritional Information

Calories 276

Net Carbs 6g

Fats 21g

Protein 19g

Fiber 2g

Baked Chicken and Avocado

Ingredients

8 pcs. chicken fillets, precooked and shredded

2 large ripe avocados, cut thin

1 onion, cut into strips

1 bell pepper, cut into strips

1 cup sour cream

1 cup cheddar cheese

1 tbsp. Sriracha sauce

salt and pepper to taste

Directions

1. Set oven at 350F
2. Grease a baking dish and lay the avocado slices on top. Set aside
3. Sauté the onion and bell pepper in a pan until it caramelizes.
4. Place the shredded chicken in a bowl and add the reset of the ingredients, including the caramelized veggies (except the avocado slices).
5. Scoop the mixture on top of the avocado slices and then place in the oven to bake for 20 minutes.
6. Serve warm.

Serves 6

Nutritional Information

Calories 549

Net Carbs 13g

Fats 40g

Protein 39g

Fiber 7g

Coco Shrimps and Chili Dip

Ingredients

12 pcs. large shrimps, peeled and deveined

1 ½ cup coconut shreds, unsweetened

¼ cup coconut flakes

6 tbsp. mayonnaise

3 tbsp. coconut milk

1 egg yolk

olive oil for frying

For the dip

4 tbsp. mayonnaise

2 tsp. chili garlic sauce

1 tsp. lime juice

Directions

1. Pat the shrimp dry set aside.
2. Combine the coconut shreds, coconut flakes, mayo, coconut milk, and egg yolk. Stir well.
3. Place the shrimps with the coconut mixture. Make sure that the shrimps are well-coated with the mixture.
4. Heat oil in the pan and fry the shrimps until golden brown.
5. Whisk all the ingredients of the dip in a small bowl. Serve alongside with the shrimps.

Serves 2

Nutritional Information

Calories 670

Net Carbs 7g

Fats 60g

Protein 11g

Fiber 3g

Slow-Cooked Spicy Chicken Soup

Ingredients

4 pcs boneless chicken fillet

4 pcs. bacon strips

1 small onion, sliced thin

1 bell pepper, sliced thin

½ tbsp. fresh thyme

½ tbsp. garlic, minced

½ tbsp. coconut flour

½ cup low-sodium chicken stock

¼ cup coconut milk, unsweetened

1 ½ tbsp. tomato paste

1 ½ tbsp. lemon juice

1 tbsp. butter

salt and pepper to taste

Directions

1. Place the butter in the middle of the slow cooker.
2. Add the onion and bell pepper slices at the bottom and then top with the chicken fillet
3. Chop the bacon and sprinkle on top of the chicken.
4. Add the rest of the ingredients (liquids last) and then cover and cook on low for 6 hours.
5. Uncover after 6 hours and break the chicken before service.
6. Serve with a spoon full of sour cream on top.

Makes 4

Nutritional Information

Calories 396

Net Carbs 7g

Fats 21g

Protein 41g

Fiber 2g

Sausage and Cheese Bombs

Ingredients

12. oz. pork sausage

¾ cup sharp cheddar cheese, shredded

12 mozzarella cheese cubes

Directions

1. Crumble the sausage and combine with the shredded cheese in a bowl.

2. Divide into 12 patties and place 1 mozzarella cube at the center of each patty.

3. Cover the cheese with the meat and create a ball.

4. Heat your fryer up to 375 and fry the meat balls until golden brown.

5. Serve with Atkins-friendly marinara sauce on the side.

Makes 12 balls

Nutritional Information

Calories 173

Net Carbs 1g

Fats 14g

Protein 10g

Fiber 0g

Homemade Chicken Nuggets

Ingredients

1 boneless chicken fillet, cooked and cut into cubes

2 tbsp. almond flour

½ tsp. baking powder

¼ cup parmesan cheese, grated

1 organic egg

1 tbsp. water

Directions

1. In a bowl, combine together the almond flour, baking powder, and parmesan.

2. Crack the egg in the bowl, pour the water and whisk the ingredients together.

3. Place the cooked chicken cubes in the batter and coat them well.

4. Heat your fryer up to 375 and fry the nuggets for 5 minutes or until golden brown.

Serves 2

Nutritional Information

Calories 166

Net Carbs 2g

Fats 8g

Protein 15g

Fiber 1g

Zucchini and Mascarpone Rolls

Ingredients

1 large zucchini cut thin using a mandolin

6 oz. mascarpone cheese

1 tsp. dill, dried

1 tsp. mint, dried

Salt and pepper to taste

1 tbsp. melted butter

Directions

1. Brush the zucchini slices with the melted butter and season with salt and pepper

2. Heat your grill and place the zucchini. Cook for 2 minutes on each side.

3. In a bowl, combine the mascarpone, dill, and mint and whisk well.

4. Equally scoop the mascarpone mixture on top of the grilled zucchini and spread.

5. Roll the zucchini and secure with toothpicks. Serve and consume immediately.

Serves 2

Nutritional Information

Calories 186

Net Carbs 3g

Fats 14g

Protein 13g

Fiber 1g

Vegetarian Cauli Rice

Ingredients

4 cups cauliflower florets

1 small onion, diced

2 cloves of garlic, minced

1 ½ tsp. garlic powder

1 ½ tsp. cumin

1 ½ tsp. chili powder

salt to taste

1 tbsp. ghee

1 cup cheddar cheese, shredded

4 tbsp. sour cream

Directions

1. Heat the ghee on a skillet over medium fire.
2. Add the onions into the hot pan and sauté for 3 minutes.
3. While waiting for the onions to cook, place the cauli florets in a food processor and pulse until they are chopped.
4. Throw in the garlic into pan and sauté for another half a minute.
5. Add the chopped cauli into the pan, along with the garlic powder, cumin, chili powder, and season with salt.
6. Cook the cauli for 12-15 minutes or until tender.
7. Turn off the heat and transfer the cauli rice into serving bowls.
8. Top with the shredded cheese and sour cream while hot.

Makes 2

Nutritional Information

Calories 618

Net Carbs 17g

Fats 48g

Protein 27g

Fiber 27g

Vegetarian-Friendly Burger Patties

Ingredients

2 cups Brussels sprouts

3 organic eggs

1 cup parmesan cheese, grated

1 ½ goat cheese

½ cup green onion, chopped

1/3 cup almond flour

1 cup parmesan cheese

1 ½ goat cheese

salt and pepper to taste

Directions

1. Thoroughly wash the Brussels sprouts and place in the food processor to shred into pieces.

2. Transfer the Brussels sprouts in a bowl and add the parmesan cheese and almond flour into the bowl. Season with salt and pepper.

3. In another bowl, whisk the eggs and the pour over the Brussels sprouts mixture. Combine well using your hands.

4. Create burger patties, about 4 oz. each and then fry on a greased cast iron skillet for about 2 minutes on each side, or until crispy.

Serves 4-5

Nutritional Information

Calories 182

Net Carbs 7g

Fats 11g

Protein 14g

Fiber 3g

Chicken Alfredo Pizza

Ingredients

½ cup left over chicken, shredded

¾ cup broccoli florets, chopped and steamed

1 cup pizza cheese mix, shredded

1 cup mozzarella cheese, shredded

¼ cup mascarpone cheese

1 tbsp. heavy cream

2 cloves of garlic, minced

salt and pepper to taste

1 tbsp. garlic infused olive oil

2 tbsp. ghee

Directions

1. Heat the garlic infused olive oil in a non-stick pan over medium heat.

2. Sprinkle the pizza cheese mix on top of the pan, allow the cheese to melt while forming it into a circle (this will be your crust).

3. Add the mozzarella cheese on the pan next and then cook for 5 minutes or until you get a crispy crust. Transfer into a pan and set aside.

4. Using the same pan, add the rest of the ingredients except the chicken and broccoli and cook for 5 minutes.

5. Pour half of the prepared alfredo sauce on top of the pizza crust and set aside.

6. Place the pan back onto the stove and add the steamed broccoli into the pan and stir for a minute.

7. Add the cheesy broccoli on top of the pizza along with the shredded roasted chicken.

8. Serve immediately.

Serves 2-3

Nutritional Information

Calories 386

Net Carbs 5.0g

Fats 27.8g

Protein 29.8g

Chicken Cordon Bleu

Ingredients

1.5 lb. chicken fillet, cut in cubes

150g ham steak, cubes

½ cup Swiss cheese, shredded

½ cup heavy cream, softened

½ cup cream cheese

½ tsp. garlic powder

salt and pepper to taste

Directions

1. Set oven at 350F.
2. Place the chicken cubes first at the bottom of an oven-safe dish.
3. Season with salt, pepper, and garlic powder.
4. Top with ham cubes and sprinkle with the Swiss cheese on top.
5. Place the cream cheese in the microwave and zap for 10 seconds. Add the heavy cream into the bowl with the melted cream cheese and stir.
6. Pour the cream mixture on top of the dish.
7. Place in the oven to cook for 40 minutes.
8. Serve hot.

Serves 5

Nutritional Information

Calories 486

Net Carbs 4g

Fats 30g

Protein 38g

Fiber 0g

Level-Up Spinach Salad

Ingredients

2 tbsp. organic butter

1 small onion, sliced thin

3 cups baby spinach

2 organic eggs, cooked hard boiled

2 bacon strips, cooked and chopped

4 tbsp. slivered almonds

4 tbsp. gorgonzola cheese

For the dressing

2 tbsp. extra virgin olive oil

2 tbsp. balsamic vinegar

salt and pepper to taste

Directions

1. Heat the butter in a pan over medium fire.

2. Add the onions, season with salt and pepper and cook for 15 minutes, or until the onions caramelize.

3. While waiting for the onions to cook, prepare the dressing by whisking all the ingredients in a bowl. Set aside.

4. Also prepare the salad by adding the spinach to the bowl and then top with the sliced hard boiled eggs, cheese, almonds, caramelized onion, and bacon.

5. Drizzle with the dressing and toss to incorporate all the ingredients.

Serves 2

Nutritional Information

Calories 607

Net Carbs 13g

Fats 52g

Protein 20g

Fiber 2.6g

Spicy Bacon-Wrapped Dogs

Ingredients

1 tbsp. ghee

1 onion, chopped

1 red bell pepper, chopped

1 pc. jalapeno, seeds removed and chopped

4 pcs. beef hot dogs

4 bacon strips

3 cheddar cheese slices

Directions

1. Heat the ghee on a non-stick pan over medium fire.

2. Add the onions, bell peppers and chopped jalapeno and sauté for 4 minutes. Remove from the pan and set aside

3. Wrap the hotdog with a bacon strips and secure with a toothpick. And cook in the same pan where the peppers were cooked.

4. Fry the dogs for 5 minutes or until crispy on both sides.

5. Lay the cheese slices on top of the cooking hotdogs and cover for 30 seconds to cook, or until the cheese melts.

6. Serve the hotdogs with the sautéed peppers on the side.

Serves 2-4

Nutritional Information

Calories 349

Net Carbs 8g

Fats 29g

Protein 14g

Chicken and Cucumber Salad

Ingredients

1 cucumber, sliced thin using a mandolin

2 boneless chicken thighs

1 small green apple, chopped

½ onion, chopped

2 tbsp. organic butter

¾ cup mayonnaise

2 tbsp. mustard

½ tsp. oregano, dried

¼ tsp. cayenne pepper

salt and pepper to taste

Directions

1. Melt the butter in a non-stick pan over medium fire.

2. Add the onions into the pan and sauté for 5-6 minutes. Set aside.

3. Season the chicken with salt and pepper and cook into the same pan. Allow the chicken to rest for at least 3 minutes before cutting into cubes. Place the fridge to chill for 30 minutes.

4. Add the mayo, dried oregano, and cayenne into a salad bowl and whisk together. Add the chicken cubes, sautéed onions, cucumber slices, and apples into the bowl and toss together.

5. Serve immediately.

Serves 2-3

Nutritional Information

Calories 502

Net Carbs 12g

Fats 41g

Protein 19g

Fiber 5.0g

Pizza on Lettuce Rolls

Ingredients

6 pcs. Romaine lettuce leaves

3 tbsp. mayonnaise

6 slices of provolone cheese

6 slices salami

6 slices pepperoni

6 slice ham

Directions

1. Lay the lettuce leaves on a serving plate.

2. Spread the mayonnaise on top of the leaves and layer with the cheese, salami, pepperoni, and ham.

3. Carefully roll the leaves and secure with a toothpick.

4. Serve and immediately.

Serves 2

Nutritional Information

Calories 592

Net Carbs 6g

Fats 46g

Protein 37g

Fiber 1.1g

Stir Fried Beef

Ingredients

1 tbsp. olive oil

12 oz. sirloin steak, cut into strips

1 onion, chopped

2 cloves of garlic, crushed

1 cup cherry tomatoes, quartered

1 red bell pepper chopped

2 tsp. ginger, grated

4 tbsp. organic apple cider vinegar

salt and pepper to taste

Directions

1. Drizzle the olive oil on a non-stick pan and heat over medium fire.

2. Season the sirloin with salt and pepper and sear onto the hot oil for 4 minutes on each side.

3. While waiting, whisk the ginner and apple cider together and pour over the steak in the pan.

4. Add the chopped onion, garlic, bell pepper, and cherry tomatoes with the beef and reduce the fire into low.

5. Cover the pan and allow to simmer for 5 minutes.

6. Turn off the heat and then allow the beef to rest for 5 minutes before serving.

Serves 2

Nutritional Information

Calories 359

Net Carbs 10g

Fats 19g

Protein 39g

Bacon and Cheese Melt

Ingredients

8 pcs. string mozzarella cheese sticks

8 strips of bacon

olive oil for frying

Directions

1. Preheat your deep fryer to 350F.

2. Wrap a cheese stick with one strip of bacon and secure with a toothpick. Repeat until you've used all the bacon and cheese.

3. Deep fry the cheese sticks in the fryer for 3 minutes.

4. Remove and place on top of a paper towel.

5. Serve with leafy green salad on the side.

Serves 2

Nutritional Information

Calories 590

Net Carbs 0g

Fats 50g

Protein 34g

Shrimp and Avocado Salad

Ingredients

12 oz. shrimp, peel removed and deveined

1 ripe avocado, peeled, cored, and cut into cubes

3 cups baby spinach

1 tomato, chopped

¼ cup green onions, chopped

¼ cup fresh cilantro, chopped

For the marinade

4 tbsp. olive oil

2 tbsp. lime juice

salt and pepper to taste

¼ tsp. garlic powder

¼ tsp. chili powder

Directions

1. In a bowl, whisk all the ingredients for the marinade.

2. Add the shrimps into the bowl and toss. Allow to marinate for 30 minutes in the fridge.

3. When the shrimps are ready, heat a non-stick pan over medium fire. Throw in the shrimp and cook for 2 minutes on each side.

4. Toss together the avocado cubes, baby spinach, chopped tomatoes, green onions, and cilantro on a bowl.

5. Top with the cooked shrimp and drizzle with an additional 1 tbsp. of olive oil.

Serves 2

Nutritional Information

Calories 428

Net Carbs 15.1g

Fats 22.8g

Protein 42.5g

Fiber 8.5g

Cheesy Cauli Mash with Bacon

Ingredients

4 cups cauliflower florets, chopped

3 tbsp. heavy cream

¼ tsp. garlic powder

salt and pepper to taste

4 bacon strips, cooked and chopped

1 cup cheddar cheese, shredded

Directions

1. In an oven-safe bowl, mix the chopped cauli florets, heavy cream, butter, and season with the garlic powder, salt, and pepper.

2. Place the bowl in the microwave and cook on high for 20 minutes or until the cauliflower is soft.

3. Pour the cooked cauliflower into a food processor and add the bacon and cheddar cheese.

4. Pulse until you achieve a smooth consistency.

5. Serve with a dab on of butter on top.

Serves 3

Nutritional Information

Calories 590

Net Carbs 6g

Fats 51g

Protein 22g

Fiber 5.0g

Breadless Cheeseburger

Ingredients

½ lb. ground beef

½ onion, chopped

1 tsp. salt

1 tsp. pepper

4 slices American cheddar

4 bacon strips, cooked and chopped

4 pcs. butter or romaine lettuce leaves

4 tbsp. mayonnaise

Directions

1. Heat a cast iron skillet over medium heat. Add the ground beef and sauté with the onions. Cook until the beef is no longer pink.

2. Season the beef with the garlic powder, salt, and pepper.

3. Reduce the heat to low and then top the beef with the slices of cheese. Cover and cook for 3 minutes, or until the cheese has melted

4. Scoop the cooked "burger patties" on the top of the lettuce leaves and dollop mayonnaise on top.

5. Serve immediately.

Serves 2

Nutritional Information

Calories 224

Net Carbs 3.2g

Fats 7.1g

Protein 34.8g

Fiber 0.9g

Trio Queso Quesadilla

Ingredients

¼ cup pepper jack cheese, shredded

¼ cup sharp cheddar cheese, shredded

1 cup mozzarella cheese, cheese

2 tbsp. coconut flour

1 organic egg

½ tsp. garlic powder

1 tbsp. almond milk, unsweetened

Directions

1. Set the oven at 350F

2. Microwave the mozzarella in the microwave until it starts to melt.

3. Allow the mozzarella to cool before adding the coconut flour, egg, garlic power, and milk.

4. Stir well until you achieve a dough-like consistency.

5. Place the dough in between two parchment papers and roll flat.

6. Remove the top parchment paper, transfer the dough on a baking sheet, and place in the oven to bake for 10 minutes.

7. Take out from the oven and allow to cool for a few minutes before topping with the cheeses on one half of the prepared tortilla.

8. Fold in half and place back in the oven to cook for 5 minutes or until the cheeses has melted.

Serves 1

Nutritional Information

Calories 977

Net Carbs 12g

Fats 73g

Protein 63g

Baked Cheesy Zucchini

Ingredients

2 pcs. zucchini, peeled and grated

¼ cup parmesan cheese, grated

½ cup mozzarella cheese, grated

1 clove of garlic

2 organic eggs

3 tbsp. organic butter (separate 1 tbsp.)

1 tsp. salt

Directions

1. Place the grated zucchini in a bowl and season with salt. Let it rest for 25 minutes.

2. Set oven at 400F

3. After the zucchini has rested for 25 mins. place it in the middle of a dishtowel and squeeze out the liquid from it. Set aside.

4. Heat the 2 tbsp. of butter on a pan and sauté the garlic for about a minute. Add the parmesan cheese and then throw in the zucchini to the pan and cook for 6 minutes. Stir occasionally.

5. Transfer into an oven-safe dish and then sprinkle with the grated mozzarella.

6. Bake in the oven for 10 minutes or until the cheese has melted.

7. While waiting for the zucchini to bake, fry the eggs using the remaining 1 tbsp. of butter.

8. Remove the zucchini from the oven when done baking and serve topped with the butter-fried egg.

Serves 2

Nutritional Information

Calories 552

Net Carbs 10g

Fats 42g

Protein 37g

Roast Chicken and Pepper Salad

Ingredients

1.5 lbs. boneless chicken thighs

1 onion, roughly chopped

1 large bell pepper, cut in half and seeded

¼ cup cilantro leaves

1 romaine lettuce

For the dressing

1 tbsp. lime juice

¼ cup mayonnaise

¼ cup sour cream

2 tbsp. olive oil

salt and pepper to taste

Directions

1. Set oven at 350F.
2. Lay the chicken thighs and onions on a baking sheet lined with foil and greased.
3. Drizzle the chicken with olive oil and season with salt and pepper.
4. Place the chicken in the oven to bake for 20 minutes. When done baking, remove from the oven and let it sit for 10 minutes.
5. Char the bell peppers while waiting for the chicken to bake. Slice into strips when done grilling.
6. In a salad bowl, whisk together the ingredients for the dressing. Add the lettuce into the bowl.
7. Top the salad with the cubed baked chicken with onions, and bell pepper on top.

8. Serve immediately.

Servings 4

Nutritional Information

Calories 349

Net Carbs 7g

Fats 16g

Protein 42g

Fiber 3g

Crab Sushi

Ingredients

1 ½ cup cauliflower florets, chopped

½ cup softened cream cheese

¾ cup crab meat, cooked

3 tbsp. mayonnaise

1 tbsp. Sriracha

1 pc. Nori wrapper

Directions

1. Pulse the cauliflower florets in a food processor and chop and until you achieve a rice-like texture.

2. Transfer the chopped cauli in a microwavable container and zap 5 minutes on high or until the vegetable is cooked.

3. Add the cream cheese with the hot cauli and stir. Place the mixture in the fridge and let it cool for an hour.

4. Place the nori wrapper on top of a sushi mat and spread the cauli mixture over it. Remember to leave a 1-inch border.

5. Meanwhile, combine all the remaining ingredients in a bowl and then scoop the crab mixture in the middle of the cauli flower rice.

6. Roll the sushi and cut into 6-8 pcs.

Serves 1

Nutritional Information

Calories 446

Net Carbs 23.4g

Fats 35.5g

Protein 10.4g

Fiber 3.8g

Sweet, Salty, and Savory Crepe

Ingredients

3 organic eggs

½ cup softened cream cheese

½ tbsp. stevia

½ tsp. cinnamon powder

4 slices ham

4 slices deli turkey

1 cup Swiss cheese, grated

2 tbsp. organic butter (divided into 2)

Directions

1. Place the first four ingredients in a food processor and pulse until you achieve a nice batter. Set aside and let it rest for 5 minutes.

2. Melt the butter on a non-stick pan over medium-high fire and scoop a heaping tablespoon of the batter into the pan. Move the pan side to side to create a crepe. Cook each side for 2 minutes.

3. Assemble the crepe by topping one side with 1 slice of ham, 1 slice of deli turkey, and sprinkle with the Swiss cheese.

4. Place another crepe on top and do the same procedure.

5. Using the same pan, melt the remaining butter and then place the stacked crepe in it. Cover and allow to cook for 2 minutes before flipping the crepe. You're done cooking when the cheese is starting to melt.

6. Serve warm.

Serves 2

Nutritional Information

Calories 825

Net Carbs 6g

Fats 67g

Protein 57g

No-Sweat Spinach Salad

Ingredients

4 cups baby spinach

4 strips of bacon, cooked and crumbled

4 tbsp. blue cheese, crumbled

¼ cup macadamia nuts, chopped

½ onion, sliced thin

¼ cup vinaigrette

Directions

1. Clean the baby spinach thoroughly and dry.
2. Place in on a salad bowl.
3. Sprinkle the blue cheese, bacon, and nuts on top.
4. Add the onions and then drizzle with vinaigrette.

Serves 4

Nutritional Information

Calories 690

Net Carbs 16.5g

Fats 66.9g

Protein 13.9g

Fiber 6.7g

Zesty Herbed Chicken

Ingredients

2 pcs boneless chicken thighs

2 tbsp. fresh parsley, chopped

½ tsp. dried oregano

4 tbsp. lemon juice

1 tbsp. olive oil

salt and pepper to taste

Directions

1. Sprinkle the lemon juice on the chicken and season with salt and pepper.

2. Heat the olive oil on a cast iron skillet over medium-high heat and then add the chicken thighs. Cook for 4-5 minutes on each side.

3. Season with oregano and turn of the heat.

4. Transfer the chicken to a serving plate and garnish with fresh parsley on top

Makes 2

Nutritional Information

Calories 469

Net Carbs 1.2g

Fats 22.9g

Protein 61.1g

Salmon Burgers

Ingredients

1 14.oz can cooked salmon flakes in water

2 organic eggs

1 cup gluten-free bread crumbs

1 small onion, chopped

1 tbsp. fresh parsley, chopped

3 tbsp. mayonnaise

2 tsp. lemon juice

salt to taste

1 tbsp. olive oil

1 tbsp. ghee

Directions

1. Crack the eggs in a bowl and use a hand mixer to whisk them until fluffy.

2. Add the bread crumbs in the bowl with the egg and combine well.

3. Add the onions, parsley, and mayonnaise and mix again.

4. Add the salmon flakes, and drizzle the lemon juice, and olive oil. Season with salt and stir again.

5. Divide the mixture into 4 parts and then create patties using your hands.

6. Heat the ghee on a cast iron skillet over medium-high fire and fry the patties until golden brown.

7. Serve with salad on the side.

Makes 4 Patties

Nutritional Information

Calories 281

Net Carbs 9.1g

Fats 25.2g

Protein 6.2g

Fiber 0.8g

Chicken Pesto Salad

Ingredients

2 cups cooked chicken, chopped

2 tbsp. organic pesto sauce

¼ cup mayonnaise

1 pc. celery, chopped

½ onion, chopped

2 tbsp. fresh parsley, chopped

salt and pepper to taste

Directions

1. Combine the chicken and the pesto sauce and mayonnaise in a bowl. Stir well.

2. Throw in the celery, onion, parsley, season with salt and pepper, and mix well.

3. Serve with fresh lettuce.

Serves 6

Nutritional Information

Calories 406

Net Carbs 10.8g

Fats 20.6g

Protein 42.7g

Fiber 1.0g

Hot Peri-Peri Chicken on Green Salad

Ingredients

2 cups baby spinach

½ boneless chicken thighs, cut into strips

1 tbsp. hot peri-peri sauce

½ ripe avocado, sliced thin

1 strip of bacon, cooked and crumbled

Directions

1. Cook the bacon first and then use the same pan to cook the bacon to fry the chicken. Place the chicken on the pan and cook for 1 minute on one side and then cook the other side for 5-6 minutes.

2. Place the baby spinach on a salad bowl and then top with the avocado and cooked chicken strips.

3. Sprinkle with the bacon crumbles and drizzle with the hot peri-peri sauce.

Serves 1

Nutritional Information

Calories 325

Net Carbs 10.8g

Fats 22g

Protein 23.9g

Fiber 8.1g

Mediterranean Chicken

Ingredients

1 whole free-range chicken, chopped into pieces

1 tsp. capers, chopped

4 ripe tomatoes, chopped

½ cup olives, chopped

½ tsp. red pepper flakes

salt and pepper to taste

2 tbsp. olive oil

Directions

1. Set the oven at 350F.

2. In a large baking dish combine the capers, tomatoes, olives, pepper flakes and olive oil. Season with salt and pepper and stir.

3. Add the chicken at the center and place in the oven to cook for an hour.

4. Serve warm.

Serves 2-3

Nutritional Information

Calories 205

Net Carbs 12g

Fats 18.2g

Protein 2.5g

Fiber 4.2g

Turkey Meatballs

Ingredients

1 lbs. turkey, ground

1 pc. organic egg

3 oz. mozzarella cheese, cubed

1 pc. green onion, chopped

2 pcs. sun-dried tomatoes, chopped

2 pcs. clove of garlic, minced

1tbsp. fresh cilantro, chopped

½ tsp. cumin powder

1 pc. shallot, chopped

salt and pepper to taste

Directions

1. Set the oven 350F.

2. In a bowl, combine the ground turkey green onions, sun-dried tomatoes, minced garlic, cilantro, cumin, and shallots. Season with salt and pepper. Combine the ingredients using your hands.

3. Form the mixture into meatballs and flatten them to create patties. Place a mozzarella cub at the center of the patty and form again into a bowl.

4. Transfer the meatballs on a baking sheet lined with parchment paper and place in the oven to bake for 30 minutes.

5. Serve warm.

Serves 2-4

Nutritional Information

Calories 509

Net Carbs 1.8g

Fats 19.1g

Protein 78.7g

Baked Glazed Salmon

Ingredients

2 pcs. salmon fillets

For the glaze:

1 tbsp. sweet mustard

1 tbsp. Dijon mustard

1 tbsp. lemon juice

½ tsp. chili flakes

1 tsp. sage

salt to taste

1 tbsp. olive oil

Directions

1. Set the oven at 350F.
2. In a bowl whisk all the ingredients for the glaze.
3. Place the salmon fillets on a baking sheet lined with parchment paper and brush the salmon fillets with the glaze.
4. Place in the oven to bake for 20 minutes. Serve warm.

Serves 2

Nutritional Information

Calories 379

Net Carbs 4.3g

Fats 24.9g

Protein 35.5g

Asian-Flavored Steak

Ingredients

4 pcs.

For the glaze marinade:

½ tsp. sesame oil

½ tsp. chili flakes

1 tsp. ginger, grated

½ cup low-sodium soy sauce

2 pcs. green onions

Directions

1. Combine all the ingredients for the marinade in a large bowl and whisk well.
2. Place the steaks in the bowl and marinate for at least 45 minutes.
3. Heat the grill on high and cook the steaks for 5 minutes on each side, or depending on your liking.

Serves 4

Nutritional Information

Calories 531

Net Carbs 4.7g

Fats 13.7g

Protein 94.4g

Curry-Spiced Salad

Ingredients

2 boneless chicken thighs, cooked and diced

2 celery stalks, diced

¼ cup carrots, minced

¼ cup roasted almonds, chopped

¼ green onions, sliced

For the dressing:

1 tsp. curry powder

3 oz. mayonnaise

3 oz. sour cream

¼ tsp. stevia

salt and pepper to taste

Directions

1. Combine all the ingredients for the dressing, whisk and set aside.

2. Place all the ingredients for the salad in a bowl, drizzle with the prepared dressing, and toss.

Serves 2

Nutritional Information

Calories 549

Net Carbs 17.1g

Fats 33.5g

Protein 45.2g

Fiber 2.5g

Eggs Benedict

Ingredients

8 organic eggs

2 egg yolks

8 strips of bacon, cooked

2 cups baby spinach

1 juice of lemon

1 tbsp. water

1 cup melted butter

¼ tsp. salt

½ tsp. pepper

½ tsp. Worcestershire sauce

Directions

1. Prepare a double boiler and medium-low fire. In the top pot, combine the yolks, lemon juice, Worcestershire sauce, pepper and a tablespoon of water. Stir well and set the sauce aside.

2. Gradually add the melted butter in the pot.

3. Meanwhile, crack an egg in a mug and zap in the microwave for a minute. Do the same thing with the rest of the 7 eggs.

4. Place the baby spinach on a serving plate and top with the chopped Canadian bacon, the microwaved eggs and drizzle with the sauce.

Serves 2

Nutritional Information

Calories 252

Net Carbs 6.4g

Fats 53.6g

Protein 15g

Fiber 1.2g

Leftover Meat Salad

Ingredients

1 cup left-over meat (chicken or pork), shredded

2 cups iceberg lettuce

1 tbsp. mayonnaise

2 tbsp. sour cream

salt and pepper to taste

Directions

1. Whisk the mayo and sour cream in a salad bowl.
2. Add the lettuce to the bowl along with the shredded meat.
3. Season with salt and pepper and toss.
4. Serve immediately.

Serves 1

Nutritional Information

Calories 252

Net Carbs 6.4g

Fats 53.6g

Protein 15g

Fiber 1.2g

Dinner Recipes

Baked Cheesy Meatballs

Ingredients

1 lb. ground beef (lean)

2 white onion

1 cup grated Cheddar cheese

4 oz. Gruyere cheese

1 egg

1.5 tsp. nutmeg

1.5 tsp. allspice

sea salt and freshly black pepper to taste

butter for greasing

Directions

1. Preheat oven to 350F.
2. In a greased frying pan, sauté onions until translucent. Remove from heat, and let cool.
3. In a food processor mince the Gruyere cheese. Set aside.
4. In a mixing bowl, whisk egg with grated Cheddar cheese. Add the spices, salt, and pepper and mix.
5. Add in onions and Gruyere cheese. Mix well until smooth.
6. Add the beef and mix until all ingredients are combined well.
7. Divide meat mixture and roll each piece into a ball.
8. Place the meatballs on a cookie sheet, and bake in preheated oven about 20 minutes. Serve hot.

Servings: 6

Cooking Times

Total Time: 35 minutes

Nutrition Facts (per serving)

Calories 385

Fat 29,05g

Carbs 4,79g

Fiber 0,91g

Protein 25,25g

Chicken & Endive Casserole

Ingredients

1 endive head, cut into wide strips

1 1/2 lbs. skinless boneless chicken thighs

1 Tbsp. dried oregano

2 cups chopped onions

4 celery stalks, chopped

4 garlic cloves, chopped

1 cup diced tomatoes in juice

2 Tbsp. olive oil

8 cups water

Directions

1. In a large saucepan heat oil over medium-high heat.

2. Sprinkle the chicken with salt, pepper, and oregano. Add chicken in a saucepan. Mix in onions, celery and garlic. Sauté until vegetables begin to soften, about 4-5minutes.

3. Stir in tomatoes. Add broth; bring to boil. Reduce heat to medium; simmer until vegetables and chicken are tender, about 15 minutes.

4. Add endive hearts; simmer until wilted, about 3 minutes. Season with salt and pepper.

5. Ladle into bowls and serve hot.

Servings: 6

Cooking Times

Total Time: 40 minutes

Nutrition Facts (per serving)

Calories 144,

Fat 7,21g

Carbs 9,94g

Fiber 2,05g

Protein 9,89g

Creamy Smoked Turkey Salad with Almonds

Ingredients

<u>Salad ingredients:</u>

2 cups diced, cooked smoked turkey breast

1/4 cup sliced almonds

1/2 cup diced celery

1/4 cup sliced green onions

1/4 cup shredded cabbage

<u>Dressing ingredients:</u>

4 oz. mayonnaise

2 oz. sour cream

2 drops sweet liquid Splenda

1 tsp. curry powder

Salt and pepper to taste

Directions

1. In a bowl, combine sour cream and mayonnaise and whisk until smooth. Add the spices and continue to whisk until smooth.
2. In a big bowl, combine all salad ingredients and the dressing and toss well. Serve and enjoy!

Note: *You can make the dressing a day ahead of time, and store in the fridge to let the flavors meld.*

Servings: 4

Cooking Times: 10 minutes

Nutrition Facts (per serving)

Calories 235

Fat 17,65g

Carbs 10,99g

Fiber 1,65g

Protein 9,84g

Herb Baked Salmon Fillets

Ingredients

2 lbs. salmon fillets

1/2 cup chopped fresh mushrooms

1/2 cup chopped green onions

4 oz. butter

4 Tbsp. coconut oil

1/2 cup tamari soy sauce

1 tsp. minced garlic

1/4 tsp. thyme

1/2 tsp. rosemary

1/4 tsp. tarragon

1/2 tsp. ground ginger

1/2 tsp. basil

1 tsp. oregano leaves

Directions

1. Preheat oven to 350 degrees F. Line a large baking pan with foil.

2. Cut salmon filet in pieces. Put the salmon into the ziploc bag with the tamari sauce, sesame oil and spices sauce mixture. Refrigerate the salmon and marinade it for 4 hours.

3. Put the salmon in a baking pan and bake fillets for 10-15 minutes.

4. Melt the butter. Add the chopped fresh mushrooms and green onion to it, and mix. Remove the salmon from the oven, and pour the butter mixture over the salmon fillets, making sure each fillet gets covered.

5. Bake for about 10 minutes more. Serve immediately.

Servings: 6

Cooking Times

Inactive Time: 4 hours

Total Time: 35 minutes

Nutrition Facts (per serving)

Calories 449

Fat 34,11g

Carbs 2,77g

Fiber 0,72g

Protein 33,19g

Beef Cabbage Parsley Soup

Ingredients

1 lb. beef shank

1/2 head cabbage, chopped

6 tsp. fresh parsley (chopped)

2 zucchini, cubed

1 tomato, quartered

1 onion, chopped

4 cloves garlic, minced

1 Tbsp. salt

1/4 tsp. ground cumin

2 Tbsp. fresh lime juice

Directions

1. In a large pot over low heat combine the beef, tomato, zucchini, onion, cabbage, garlic, 5 teaspoons parsley, salt and cumin.

2. Add water to cover and stir well. Cover lid and cook for 2 hours.

3. Remove lid, stir, and simmer for another 1 hour with lid off.

4. Just before eating, squeeze in fresh lime juice to taste and sprinkle with remaining parsley.

5. Serve hot.

Servings: 8

Cooking Times

Total Time: 2 hours and 5 minutes

Nutrition Facts (per serving)

Calories 129

Fat 2,35g

Carbs 13,28g

Fiber 2,08g

Protein 14,11g

Boneless Lamb Stew

Ingredients

2 lbs. boneless lamb meat, cubed

1 cup red onion, chopped

2 whole celery stalks, diced

4 cloves garlic, minced

1 cup tomato juice

2 Tbsp. extra virgin coconut oil

1 cup lime juice (freshly squeezed)

1 bay leaf

1 tsp. ground cinnamon

1 tsp. ground nutmeg

Fresh parsley, chopped for topping

Sea salt and freshly ground black pepper, to taste

Directions

1. Put the lamb in a glass bowl and season with the salt, pepper, cinnamon, and nutmeg. Place in refrigerator for up to 24 hours.

2. In a large casserole, heat the coconut oil over medium heat. Add pieces of lamb and brown on all sides.

3. Once browned, add the onion, garlic and celery. Cook for about five minutes, stirring often, until vegetables start to soften.

4. Add the tomato juice, lime juice and bay leaf; stir till mixture begins to boil.

5. Reduce the heat to low and cook for about 2 hours.

6. Serve hot with fresh chopped parsley.

Servings: 6

Cooking Times

Total Time: 2 hours and 10 minutes

Nutrition Facts (per serving)

Calories 250

Fat 11,82g

Carbs 6,86g

Fiber 1,67g

Protein 21,68g

Butternut Squash Soup

Ingredients

3 lbs. butternut squash

4 cloves garlic, minced

1 cup yellow onion, sliced

1 cup coconut milk

2 tsp. olive oil

1 bay leaf

2 cup water

1/2 tsp. salt and pepper (per taste)

coconut oil or olive oil for greasing

Directions

1. Preheat oven to 450° F.

2. On a greased baking sheet, place the squash and onion with half oil and salt. Roast in a single layer about 25-30 minutes.

3. Transfer the vegetables to a large saucepan with olive oil and cook over HIGH heat for 3-5 minutes. Stir often.

4. Add garlic and cook for another 30 seconds. Add the water, bay leaf and coconut milk; bring to a boil.

5. Reduce heat to MEDIUM-LOW, cover and simmer for 10 minutes more.

6. At the end, remove bay leaf and transfer squash mixture to a blender. Puree until smooth. Add salt and pepper to taste.

7. Ladle to bowls and serve hot.

Servings: 10

Cooking Times

Total Time: 55 minutes

Nutrition Facts (per serving)

Calories 120

Fat 7,12g

Carbs 12,74g

Fiber 2,3g

Protein 3,48g

Creamy Chicken Salad

Ingredients

Salad ingredients

2 cups diced, cooked chicken

1/2 cup sliced green onion

1/4 cup parsley, chopped

1/2 cup diced celery

Dressing ingredients

4 oz. mayonnaise

2 oz. blue cream cheese, softened

1 tsp. dried tarragon

1/2 tsp. dried thyme

salt and pepper to taste

Directions

1. In a bowl, whisk cream cheese and mayonnaise until smooth.
2. Add the spices and continue to whisk.
3. Combine the salad ingredients and add dressing to taste, mixing to coat all the ingredients.
4. Serve immediately.

Servings: 4

Cooking Times

Total Time: 10 minutes

Nutrition Facts (per serving)

Calories 250

Fat 12,23g

Carbs 9,77g

Fiber 0,78g

Protein 24,74g

Duck Breast with Balsamic Vinegar

Ingredients

1 lb. duck breasts

4 Tbsp. duck fat (or lark)

4 green onions (chopped)

1 tsp. fresh ginger grated

1/2 Tbsp. lime juice

Marjoram to taste

2 Tbsp. coconut oil

2 Tbsp. apple cider vinegar

salt and freshly ground pepper to taste

Directions

1. In a frying pan add 1 tablespoon coconut oil and add the duck breast. Sauté it at high heat about 3-4 minutes.

2. In a deep saucepan add the duck fat, and add the duck meat. Cook for 3 hours about. Add the chopped green onions in the last 30 minutes of the cooking process.

3. Remove green onion and duck breast from the heat, and place them in a separate dish to cool down. Sprinkle the marjoram, balsamic vinegar and the lime juice. Serve hot.

Servings: 4

Nutrition Facts (per serving)

Calories 471,

Fat 46,68g

Carbs 2,76g

Fiber 0,42g

Protein 10,11g

Hot Mexican Meatballs

Ingredients

1 lb. ground beef (92% lean)

4 oz. white onion, minced

4 oz. Monterey Jack cheese with spicy peppers

1 Tbsp. butter

3 cloves garlic

1 1 tsp. chili powder

1 1 tsp. ground cumin

1 tsp. ground coriander

1 egg

sea salt and freshly ground pepper to taste

Directions

1. Preheat oven to 350 degrees.
2. In a frying pan, sauté onions in butter until translucent. Set aside
3. Shred and mince the Monterey Jack cheese with spicy peppers. Set aside.
4. In a mixing bowl, whisk egg with ricotta cheese. Add the spices, salt, and pepper and mix.
5. Add onions and minced Monterey Jack cheese with spicy peppers. Mix well.
6. Add beef and mix until all ingredients are combined.
7. Roll the meat mix into a ball.
8. Place the meatballs on a cookie sheet, and bake about 20 minutes.
9. Serve hot.

Servings: 6

Cooking Times
Total Time: 35 minutes

Nutrition Facts (per serving)
Calories 321
Fat 25,25g
Carbs 2,94g
Fiber 0,9g
Protein 19,54g

Lamb Cutlets with Garlic Sauce

Ingredients

4 lbs. lamb cutlets

1 small head of garlic, cloves peeled

2 Tbsp. apple cider vinegar

1/2 cup water

1/4 cup extra virgin olive oil

pinch salt and black ground pepper to taste

Directions

1. Crush the garlic cloves thoroughly in a mortar. In a bowl, add the vinegar and water and mix it well with the crushed garlic. Set aside.

2. In a large frying pan, pour the olive oil and fry the lamb cutlets until nicely brown.

3. Add the garlic mixture and let it cook gently for about 10 minutes.

4. Shake the frying pan to spread the garlic mixture evenly over the lamb.

5. Season with salt and black pepper to taste. Serve.

Servings: 10

Cooking Times

Total Time: 40 minutes

Nutrition Facts (per serving)

Calories 416

Fat 28,76g

Carbs 0,16g

Fiber 0,01g

Protein 36,68g

Almond Bread

Ingredients

2 eggs

1 cup almond butter, unsalted

3/4 cup almond flour

1 Tbsp. cinnamon

1 tsp. pure vanilla extract

1/4 tsp. baking soda

2 Tbsp. liquid Stevia

1/2 tsp. sea salt

Directions

1. Preheat oven to 340F degrees.

2. In a deep bowl whisk eggs, almond butter, honey, Stevia and vanilla. Add in salt, cinnamon and baking soda. Stir until all ingredients are well combined.

3. Pour dough in a greased baking pan. Bake for 12-15 minutes.

4. Once ready, let cool on a wire rack. Slice and serve.

Servings: 8

Cooking Times

Total Time: 25 minutes

Nutrition Facts (per serving)

Calories 208

Fat 16,7g

Carbs 7,64g

Fiber 3,63g

Protein 7,7g

Slow Cooker Buffalo Chicken

Ingredients

3 Tbsp. butter

6 frozen chicken breasts

1 bottle of your favorite cayenne peppers sauce

1 cup of your favorite garlic sauce

Directions

1. Put the chicken in the bottom of your Slow Cooker. Pour the hot sauce over chicken and sprinkle ranch over top

2. Cover the lid and cook on LOW for 6 hours.

3. Once ready, add butter, and cook on LOW uncovered for one hour more. Serve hot.

Servings: 4

Cooking Time: 6 hours and 5 minutes

Nutrition Facts (per serving)

Calories 517

Fat 18,41g

Carbs 2,26g

Fiber 0,37g

Protein 80,37g

Spiced Kale "Meatballs"

Ingredients

4 Tbsp. olive oil

1 cup almond flour

1 bunch of kale leaves

1 green chili, chopped

1/4 tsp. red chili powder

1/4 tsp. turmeric powder

1 tsp. cumin seed powder

1/4 tsp. ginger, minced

black salt or salt as per taste

1 tsp. cooking soda or baking soda (optional)

water for batter

Directions

1. In a bowl, mix all the ingredients together.

2. Combine and knead the batter with your finger. The consistency should be nor too thick nor too thin. Make a kale "meatballs".

3. Heat oil in a frying pan. Place a kale "meatballs" in the hot oil one by one.

4. Fry few at a time don't cluster with too many. When they get golden color from one side, turn and cook from another side.

5. Remove the fries with slotted spoon and place over absorbent napkins.

6. Serve hot.

Servings: 8

Cooking Times

Total Time: 25 minutes

Nutrition Facts (per serving)

Calories 125

Fat 6,24g

Carbs 13,01g

Fiber 4,85g

Protein 6,04g

Spinach Soup with Almonds and Parmesan

Ingredients

1 lb. baby spinach leaves

1 leek

1 zucchini (medium)

1/4 cup parmesan cheese (grated)

4 Tbsp. olive oil

4 cups water

15 almond shivers

salt and black ground pepper to taste

Directions

1. Wash the leek and cut it into thick slices.

2. Heat the olive oil in a saucepan and cook the zucchini and leek for about 2-3 minutes.

3. Add the cleaned spinach leaves, water and a pinch of salt. Bring to the boil and let it simmer for 15 minutes.

4. Remove from the heat and place the vegetables in a food processor. Blend into a very smooth soup.

5. In a frying pan, toast the almonds. Pour the soup into bowls, sprinkle with some Parmesan cheese on top and toasted almonds.

6. Serve.

Servings: 6

Cooking Times

Total Time: 45 minutes

Nutrition Facts (per serving)

Calories 63

Fat 3,04g

Carbs 5,94g

Fiber 2,47g

Protein 4,84g

Stuffed Avocado with Tuna

Ingredients

2 ripe avocados, halved and pitted

1 can (15 oz.) solid white tuna packed in water, drained

2 Tbsp. mayonnaise

3 green onions, thinly sliced

1 Tbsp. cayenne paprika

1 red bell pepper, chopped

1 Tbsp. balsamic vinegar

1 pinch garlic salt and black pepper to taste

Directions

1. In a bowl, toss together tuna, mayonnaise, cayenne pepper, green onions, red pepper, and balsamic vinegar.

2. Season with pepper and salt, and then pack the avocado halves with the tuna mixture.

3. Ready! Serve and enjoy!

Servings: 4

Cooking Times

Total Time: 20 minutes

Nutrition Facts (per serving)

Calories 233

Fat 17,77g

Carbs 13,87g

Fiber 6,98g

Protein 7,41g

Light Cabbage Soup

Ingredients

2 1/2 cups chopped cabbage

4 garlic cloves, minced

1 Tbsp. tomato paste

1 onion, chopped

1/2 cup parsnip, chopped

1/2 cup cauliflower florets

1/2 cup chopped zucchini

1/2 tsp. basil

1/2 tsp. oregano

Salt and black pepper, to taste

4 cups water

olive oil for sautéing

Directions

1. In a frying pan, sauté onions, parsnip and garlic for 5 minutes.

2. Add in water, tomato paste, cabbage, cauliflower, basil, oregano and salt and pepper to taste.

3. Simmer for a about 5-10 minutes until all vegetables are tender. Add the zucchini and simmer for another 5 minutes.

4. Serve hot.

Servings: 4

Cooking Times

Total Time: 35 minutes

Nutrition Facts (per serving)

Calories 80

Fat 3,08g

Carbs 9,69g

Fiber 3,04g

Protein 4,62g

Oriental Shrimp Soup

Ingredients

12 oz. fresh shrimp, peeled and deveined

1 cup zucchini (medium, sliced)

1 onion, chopped

2 cloves garlic, minced

1 Tbsp. ginger, minced

1 pinch crushed red pepper

2 quarts water

1 cup celery (chopped)

2 cups cauliflower florets

2 Tbsp. soy sauce

1/4 tsp. ground black pepper

2 tsp. olive oil

Directions

1. In a large saucepan with over medium heat cook onion, garlic, ginger and crushed red pepper for 2 minutes.

2. Pour in water, cauliflower florets and celery and bring to a boil. Reduce heat, cover and simmer 5 minutes.

3. Stir in zucchini and shrimp, season with salt and pepper to taste; cover and cook 5 - 7 minutes.

4. Stir in soy sauce and pepper and serve.

Servings: 8

Cooking Times

Total Time: 25 minutes

Nutrition Facts (per serving)

Calories 107

Fat 3,08g

Carbs 7,12g

Fiber 1,6g

Protein 12,08g

Slow Cooker Beef with Dried Herbs

Ingredients

1 1/2 lbs. lean beef

2 celery ribs

1 cup beef broth

2 Tbsp. amaranth flour

2 Tbsp. almond butter

2 Tbsp. olive oil

1 tsp. mustard

2 Tbsp. fresh lemon juice

4 Tbsp. chopped parsley

salt, pepper, dried thyme, dried marjoram

Directions

1. In a bowl, toss the beef with the amaranth flour. Heat the butter and oil in a skillet; add the beef and cook, stirring, until browned.

2. In a slow cooker combine the browned beef with remaining ingredients, except lemon juice and parsley.

3. Cover and cook on LOW for 6 to 8 hours.

4. Once ready, stir in lemon juice and parsley and serve hot.

Servings: 6

Cooking Times

Total Time: 8 hours

449

Nutrition Facts (per serving)

Calories 387

Fat 31,96g

Carbs 2,56g

Fiber 0,2g

Protein 20,96g

Zucchini Soup with Crunchy Cured Ham

Ingredients

2 leeks (white part only)

12 ounces zucchinis

10 ounces summer squash

3 Tbsp. virgin olive oil

5 cups water

salt

2 slices cured ham

black pepper

Directions

1. Cut the leeks into thin slices and chop the zucchinis and summer squash into cubes.

2. In a large saucepan, heat the olive oil and add the leeks. Cook the leeks until they are soft, stirring gently.

3. Add in the chopped zucchinis and summer squash and cook them for about 5 minutes.

4. Add in water and bring to the boil for about 15 minutes.

5. Blend or process the soup in batches until smooth.

6. Season the soup to taste.

7. In a frying pan cook striped ham until crispy.

8. Divide the soup amongst the serving bowls and sprinkle with the crunchy ham strips and some black pepper.

9. Serve hot.

Servings: 4

Cooking Times

Total Time: 45 minutes

Nutrition Facts (per serving)

Calories 84

Fat 1,89g

Carbs 8,75g

Fiber 1,52g

Protein 8,54g

Salmon with a Walnut Crust

Ingredients

Walnuts (1/2 cup)

Dijon mustard (1/2 tablespoon)

Salmon filets (6 oz.)-2

Salt

Maple syrup (2 tablespoons, sugar free)

Dill (1/4 teaspoon)

Olive oil (1 tablespoon)

Directions

1. Set oven to 350 °F.
2. Put mustard, syrup and walnuts into a processor and pulse until mixture is pasty.
3. Heat oil in a pot and place the skin side down in the pan and sear for 3 minutes.
4. Top it with walnut blend and place into a lined baking dish.
5. Bake for 8 minutes.
6. Serve.

Servings: 2

Nutrition Facts (per serving)

Calories 373

Fats 43g

Protein 20 g

Fiber 1g

Cheeseburger Casserole

Ingredients

Bacon (3 slices)

Cauliflower (1 ¼ cups)

Garlic powder (1/2 teaspoon)

Ketchup (2 tablespoons, no sugar)

Mayonnaise (2 tablespoons)

Cheddar cheese (4 oz.)

Ground beef (1 lb.)

Almond flour (1/2 cup)

Psyllium Husk Powder (1 tablespoon)

Onion powder (1/2 teaspoon)

Dijon mustard (1 tablespoon)

Eggs (3)

Salt

Black pepper

Directions

1. Set oven to 350 ℉.

2. Place cauliflower into a processor and pulse until fine like rice. Add remaining dry ingredients except cheese.

3. Add beef and bacon in processor until combined and pasty.

4. Heat skillet and cook meat for 8 minutes then add to dry ingredients in bowl along with half of cheese. Stir to combine and line a baking dish with parchment paper.

5. Press mixture into dish and top with leftover cheese. Bake for 30 minutes on top rack.

6. Take from heat, cool and slice.

7. Serve.

Servings: 6

Nutrition Facts (per serving)

Calories 478

Net Carbs 3.6g

Fats 35.5g

Protein 32.2 g

Fiber 3.3g

Curried Coconut Chicken Fingers

Ingredients

Chicken thighs (24 oz., boneless with skin)

Pork rinds (1/2 cup, crushed)

Curry powder (2 teaspoons)

Garlic powder (1/4 teaspoon)

Salt

Black pepper

Egg (1)

Coconut (1/2 cup, shredded, unsweetened)

Coriander (1/2 teaspoon)

Onion powder (1/4 teaspoon)

For Dipping Sauce:

Sour cream (1/4 cup)

Mango extract (1 ½ teaspoons)

Garlic powder (1/2 teaspoon)

Cayenne powder (1/4 teaspoon)

Mayonnaise (1/4 cup)

Ketchup (2 tablespoons, sugar free)

Red pepper flakes (1 ½ teaspoons)

Ground ginger (1/2 teaspoon)

Liquid Stevia (7 drops)

Directions
1. Set oven to 400 F.
2. Beat egg in a bowl and slice chicken into strips.
3. Combine spices, pork rind and coconut in another bowl. Coat with egg and then in dry mix.

4. Place onto a lined baking sheet and bake for 15 minutes and turn over; bake for an additional 20 minutes.
5. Combine all ingredients for dipping sauce in a bowl and serve with chicken.

Servings: 6

Nutrition Facts (per serving)

Calories 494
Net Carbs 2.1g
Fats 39.4g
Protein 29.4 g
Fiber 1.2g

Slow Cooker Lamb Curry & Spinach

Ingredients

Coconut or olive oil (1/3 cup)

3 copped yellow onions

4 cloves garlic, peeled and minced

2cm piece of ginger, peeled and grated

Ground cumin (2 teaspoons)

Cayenne pepper (1 1/2 teaspoons).

Ground turmeric (1 1/2 teaspoons).

Beef stock, high quality (2 cups)

Leg of lamb, cut into 2cm cubes (53 oz.)

Salt

Baby spinach (6 cups)

Plain full-fat yogurt (2 cups)

Directions

1. In a large frying pan over medium-high heat, warm oil. Add onions and garlic, and sauté until golden, about 5 minutes. Stir in ginger, cumin, cayenne, and turmeric and sauté until fragrant, or for about 30 seconds.

2. Pour in broth scraping up the browned bits on the bottom. When broth comes to a boil, remove pan from heat.

3. Put lamb in a slow cooker, and sprinkle with 1 tbsp. salt. Add contents of frying pan. Cover and cook on high-heat setting for 4 hours or low-heat setting for 8 hours.

4. Add baby spinach to pot and cook, stirring occasionally, until spinach is wilted, about 5 minutes. Just before serving, stir in 1 1/3 cups yogurt. Season to taste with salt.

Servings: 5

Nutrition Facts (per serving)

Calories- 304

Carbs- 5.5g

Protein- 32.85g

Fats- 16.32g

Curried Madras Lamb

Ingredients

8 Fatty lamb chops

Coconut Milk (6 tablespoons)

2 cups water

Red Curry Paste (3 tablespoons)

Thai fish sauce (2 tablespoons)

Dried onion flakes (1 tablespoon)

Dried Thai or fresh red chilies (2 tablespoons)

Xylitol (1 tablespoon)

Ground cumin (1 tablespoon)

Ground coriander (1 tablespoon)

Ground cloves (1/8 teaspoon)

Ground nutmeg (1/8 teaspoon)

Ground ginger (1 tablespoon)

To Serve:

Coconut milk powder (2 tablespoons)

Red curry paste (1 tablespoons)

Xylitol (2 tablespoons)

1/4 cup cashews, roughly chopped

1/4 cup fresh cilantro, chopped

Directions

1. Place the raw lamb chops in a large slow cooker.

2. Add the 6 tbsp. coconut milk, water, 3 tbsp. red curry paste, fish sauce, onion flakes, chilies, 1 tbsp. Xylitol, cumin, coriander, cloves, nutmeg, and ginger. Cover and cook on high for about 5 hours (or low for 8).

3. Just before serving, scoop out the meat to another dish. Then whisk into the sauce the 2 tbsp. coconut milk powder, 1 tbsp. curry paste, 2 tbsp. sweetener, and 1/4 tsp. xanthan gum (if using).

4. Break the meat into pieces and stir into the sauce, along with the chopped cashews. Garnish with chopped coriander before serving

Servings: 5

Nutrition Facts (per serving)

Calories- 190
Carbs- 4g
Protein- 18g
Fats- 11g

Seafood Stew

Ingredients

Olive oil (1 tablespoon)

2 onions, diced

4 stalks celery, chopped

4 garlic cloves, minced

Dried oregano (1 teaspoon)

Ground black pepper (1/2 teaspoon)

Tomato paste (1 tablespoon)

Flour (1 tablespoon)

3 cups chicken stock

1 can tomato, onion and chili mix

1 -2 cup tomato cocktail juice

4 chicken breasts cut into bite size pieces

2 packets mixed frozen seafood, you can add extra

mussels in at the end

2 peppers (red and green)

1 jalapeno pepper, chopped

1/4cup parsley, chopped

Chili powder (1 teaspoon)

1 pinch cayenne pepper

Butter (1 tablespoon)

Directions

1. In a large pan heat the olive oil and fry onions and celery
2. Add garlic, oregano, peppercorns.
3. Stir in tomato paste and almond flour and cook another minute.

4. Add chicken stock, tomatoes and tomato juice and bring to a boil. Continue to cook for about 3-5 more minutes. Remove from heat and transfer mixture to slow cooker.
5. Add chicken and stir to combine. Cover and cook on high for 3 hours or low for 6 hours.
6. Stir in mixed bags of frozen and parsley. Cover and cook on high for 30 minutes

Servings: 5

Nutrition Facts (per serving)

Calories- 177
Carbs- 15g
 Protein- 21g
 Fats- 4g

Slow Cooker Thai Fish Curry

Ingredients

Coconut oil (1 tablespoon)

Green Thai curry paste (1/2 tablespoons)

8-10 spring onions

2 garlic cloves, crushed

1 Thai red chili, deseeded if you like, and thinly sliced

Turmeric (1 teaspoon)

Chicken stock (160ml)

1½ cups coconut milk

2.5cm piece of fresh ginger, peeled and sliced

Xylitol (2 teaspoons)

Juice of 1 lime, plus extra to taste

Fish sauce (1 teaspoon)

700g boneless, skinless white fish, such as cod, hake or halibut cut into large chunks

freshly ground black pepper

chopped coriander leaves, to serve

Directions

1. Fry Spring onions, garlic and chilies then stir in green Thai Curry Paste and then sprinkle over the turmeric.

2. Add the stock, coconut milk, ginger, Xylitol and juice from a fresh lime and season with pepper. Bring to the boil, stirring to dissolve the paste and xylitol, and then pour the mixture into the slow cooker.

3. Cover the cooker with the lid and cook on HIGH for 1 hour until the flavors are well blended. Add the fish sauce, if using, and add a little more xylitol and fresh lime juice, if you like.

4. Switch the cooker to LOW. Add the fish, re-cover and cook until the fish is cooked through and flakes easily.

5. Sprinkle with coriander and lime zest and sliced red chilies.

Servings: 5

Nutrition Facts (per serving)

Calories 312

Carbs 20g

Protein 24g

Fats 15g

Smoky Pork Cassoulet

Ingredients

1 pack bacon, fried and then crumbled

Chopped onion (2 cups)

Dried thyme (1 teaspoon)

Dried rosemary (1/2 teaspoon)

3 garlic cloves, crushed

Salt (1/2 teaspoon)

Freshly ground black pepper (1/2 teaspoon)

2 cans diced tomatoes, drained

500g boneless pork loin roast, trimmed and cut into 2cm cubes

250g smoked sausage, cut into 1cm cubes

Finely shredded fresh Parmesan cheese (8 teaspoons)

Chopped fresh flat-leaf parsley (8 teaspoons)

Directions

1. Fry bacon onion, thyme, rosemary, and garlic, then add salt, pepper, and tomatoes; bring to a boil.

2. Remove from heat.

3. Place all ingredients in the slow cooker, alternating the meat with the tomato sauce until finished. Cover and cook on low for 5 hours. Sprinkle with Parmesan cheese and parsley when cooked

Servings: 4

Nutrition Facts (per serving)

Calories- 258

Carbs- 10.8g

Protein- 27g

Fats- 12.6g

Sage and Orange Glazed Duck

Ingredients

Butter (2 tablespoons)

Swerve (1 tablespoon)

Sage (1/4 teaspoon)

Duck breast (6 oz.)

Heavy cream (1 tablespoon)

Orange extract (1/2 teaspoon)

Spinach (1 cup)

Directions

1. Use knife to score the skin of the duck and season with black pepper and salt.

2. Add Swerve and butter to a pot and cook until slightly golden then add extract and sage. Cook until butter has darkened.

3. In another pot, place chicken breast with skin side down and place over a medium flame and cook until skin is crisp.

4. Flip over and add cream to sage mixture and pour over duck. Cook until duck is done.

5. Add spinach to pot and cook until wilted.

6. Serve.

Servings: 1

Nutrition Facts (per serving)

Calories 798

Net Carbs 0g

Fats 71g

Protein 36 g

Fiber 1g

Chicken Pot Pie

Ingredients

For filling:

Bacon (5 slices)

Garlic powder (1 teaspoon)

Cream cheese (8 oz.)

Spinach (6 cups)

Salt

Chicken thighs (6, boneless and skinless)

Onion powder (1 teaspoon)

Celery seed (3/4 teaspoon)

Cheddar cheese (4 oz.)

Chicken broth (1/4 cup)

For crust:

Psyllium Husk Powder (3 tablespoons)

Eggs (1)

Cheddar cheese (1/4 cup)

Garlic powder (1/4 teaspoon)

Salt

Almond flour (1/3 cup)

Butter (3 tablespoons)

Cream cheese (1/4 cup)

471

Paprika (1/2 teaspoon)

Onion powder (1/4 teaspoon)

Black pepper

Directions

1. Cube chicken and season with black pepper and salt.

2. Set oven to 375 °F.

3. Use spices to season chicken and place into an oven proof skillet and place onto fire and cook until golden on the outside. Add bacon to pan and cook until golden.

4. Add broth to pan along with cheeses and stir to combine. Put in spinach in pan and cook until wilted.

5. Combine dry ingredients for crust in a bowl and add cheddar and cream cheese to a microwave safe dish and then add cheese and combine. Add mixture to dry ingredients and mix together.

6. Form crust, stir ingredients in pot and top with crust and use fork to pierce crust all over.

7. Bake for 15 minutes, take from oven and cool.

8. Serve.

Servings: 8

Nutrition Facts (per serving)

Calories 434

Net Carbs 3.4g

Fats 35.6g

Protein 20.4 g

Fiber 3.6g

Chicken Parmesan

Ingredients

For Chicken:

Chicken breasts (3)

Mozzarella cheese (1 cup)

Salt

Black pepper

For coating:

Flaxseed meal (1/4 cup)

Oregano (1 teaspoon)

Black pepper (1/2 teaspoon)

Garlic powder (1/2 teaspoon)

Egg (1)

Pork rinds (2.5 oz.)

Parmesan cheese (1/2 cup)

Salt (1/2 teaspoon)

Red pepper flakes (1/4 teaspoon)

Paprika (2 teaspoons)

Chicken broth (1 ½ teaspoons)

For Sauce:

Tomato sauce (1 cup, low carb)

Garlic (2 cloves)

474

Salt

Olive oil (1/2 cup)

Oregano (1/2 teaspoon)

Black pepper

Directions

1. Add flax meal, spices, pork rinds and parmesan cheese in a processor and grind until combined.

2. Pound chicken breast and whisk egg with broth in a container. Add all ingredients for sauce to a pan stir and put over a low flame to cook.

3. Dip chicken in egg and then coat with dry mixture.

4. Heat oil in a pan and fry chicken then transfer to a casserole dish. Top with sauce and mozzarella and bake for 10 minutes.

5. Serve.

Servings: 4

Nutrition Facts (per serving)

Calories 646

Net Carbs 4g

Fats 46.8g

Protein 49.3g

Fiber 2.8g

Bell Peppers Stuffed Korean Beef

Ingredients

Ground beef (1 lb.)

Spring onions (2, sliced)

Ginger (2 teaspoons, diced)

Eggs (8)

Bell peppers (2, cut in half)

Garlic (2 teaspoons, diced)

Salt

Black pepper

For Sauce:

Rice wine vinegar (1 ½ tablespoons)

Chili paste (1 tablespoon)

Apricot preserves (1/3 cup, sugar free)

Ketchup (1 tablespoon, low sugar)

Soy sauce (1 tablespoon)

Directions

1. Season beef with pepper and salt and start cooking over a medium flame until browned. Add ginger and garlic and stir together.

2. Push beef to one side and put in spring onions, cook for 2 minutes then stir together with beef. Take from flame and put aside.

3. Add all sauce ingredients to a pan and cook for 3 minutes then add half to beef.

4. Stir sauce and beef together and use to stuff peppers.

5. Set oven to 350 F and bake for 15 minutes.

6.   Top with reserved sauce and serve.

Servings: 4

Nutrition Facts (per serving)

Calories 470

Net Carbs 6.3g

Fats 35g

Protein 32.3g

Fiber 5.3g

Creamy Tarragon Chicken

Ingredients

Chicken breast (5 oz.)

Onion (1/4, sliced)

Chicken broth (1/2 cup)

Grain mustard (1 teaspoon)

Salt

Olive oil (1 tablespoon)

Mushrooms (3 oz.)

Heavy cream (1/4 cup)

Tarragon (1/2 teaspoon, dried)

Black pepper

Directions

1. Cube chicken and season with pepper and salt.

2. Heat oil in a pan and sauté chicken for 6 minutes until golden all over. Take from pan and put aside.

3. Add mushrooms and cook for 3 minutes until golden then add onion and cook for 3 minutes until soft and translucent.

4. Add broth and bring to a boil for 4 minutes then add remaining ingredients and adjust black pepper and salt to taste.

5. Return chicken to sauce in pan and cook for 5 minutes.

6. Serve.

Servings: 1

Nutrition Facts (per serving)

Calories 490

Net Carbs 5g

Fats 40g

Protein 32 g

Fiber 1g

Beanless Chili con Carne

Ingredients

Ground beef (1 lb.)

Green pepper (1, chopped)

Onion (1, chopped)

Curry powder (2 tablespoons)

Cumin (2 tablespoons)

Coconut oil (1 tablespoon)

Onion powder (1 teaspoon)

Black pepper (1 teaspoon)

Italian sausage (1 lb., spicy)

Yellow pepper (1, chopped)

Tomato sauce (16 oz.)

Chili powder (2 tablespoons)

Garlic (1 tablespoon, diced)

Butter (1 tablespoon)

Salt (1 teaspoon)

Directions

1. Heat oil and butter in a pan, heat thoroughly and add garlic, onions and bell peppers. Cook for 3 minutes then add beef and sausage.
2. Cook for 5 minutes until browned then add onion and chili powder. Stir to combine and add tomato sauce. Lower flame and cook for 20 minutes.
3. Add cumin and curry, stir and cook for 45 minutes or until chili thickens to your liking.
4. Serve.

Servings: 5

Nutrition Facts (per serving)

Calories 415

Net Carbs 6g

Fats 25g

Protein 146 g

Fiber 51g

Seared Ribeye Steak

Ingredients

Ribeye steaks (2 medium)

Salt

Black pepper

Bacon fat (3 tablespoons)

Directions

1. Set oven to 250 °F.

2. Place a wire rack over a baking sheet and place steaks on rack.

3. Use pepper and salt to season steaks and bake until steak's internal temperature is 123 °F.

4. Melt fat in a cast iron pan until it is extremely hot then transfer steaks to pot and sear on both sides.

5. Let steaks sit for a few minutes before slicing.

6. Serve.

Servings: 5

Nutrition Facts (per serving)

Calories 430

Net Carbs 0g

Fats 31.7g

Protein 30.3 g

Italian Fish Stew

Ingredients

4 200g Kingklip fish fillets

2 onions, finely chopped

4 garlic cloves, minced

2 tins peeled, chopped tomato

4 tbsp. tomato paste

250ml white wine

½ tsp. parsley, chopped

¼ tsp. dried oregano

salt and pepper to taste

½ cup olive oil

1 cup water

Directions

1. Preheat oven to 360C

2. Sauté onion and garlic on a pot then add tinned tomatoes and tomato paste and stir.

3. Pour the wine, parsley, oregano, salt, pepper, and water. Stir well and bring to a simmer.

4. Let it simmer for 10-15 minutes to reduce and thicken.

5. Meanwhile, place your fish in baking dish.

6. When sauce is nice and thick, pour it over fish and sprinkle with a little extra oregano.

7. Cover the dish with foil and place in the oven to cook for 20 minutes.

8. Take foil off and return to oven uncovered and cook for another 10 minutes.

Tip: If the sauce is a little runny when fish comes out, place sauce in another pot and put on heat to reduce a little more. Then pour back over fish.

Nutritional Info (per serving)

Calories: 315

Net Carbs: 12

Fat: 8g

Protein: 37g

Chicken Stir-Fry

Ingredients

4 chicken breasts (butterfly), marinate in egg white overnight

2 cups red pepper

2 cups mange tout

2 cups grated carrot

2 cups broccoli

2 cups almonds

2 cloves of garlic

½ tsp. ginger

2 tbsp. soya sauce

125ml chicken stock.

2 tbsp. coconut oil

Directions

1. Heat coconut oil in a pan over medium fire. Sauté the garlic and ginger until fragrant.

2. Cook the chicken breast in the oil and then add the vegetables. Toss and cook until almost done.

3. Add 2 tbsp. soya sauce and 125ml chicken stock. Allow to simmer uncovered until the broth evaporates.

Nutritional Info

Calories: 186

Net Carbs: 4g

Fat: 11g

Protein: 17g

Pan Fried Hake

Ingredients

1 tbsp. olive oil

Salt and pepper to taste

1 250g Hake fillet

fresh lemon wedges

Directions

1. Heat the olive oil in a large frying pan over medium-high heat.

2. Pat the fish dry with kitchen paper towel and then season with salt and pepper on both sides.

3. Fry the fish for about 4-5 minutes on each side, depending on their thickness, or until they have a golden crust and the flesh flakes away easily with a fork.

Nutritional Info (per serving)

Calories: 170

Net Carbs: 7g

Fat: 8g

Protein: 18g

Creamed Spinach

Ingredients

2 cups spinach

½ small onion, chopped

¼ cup water

½ stock cube

1 clove of garlic, chopped

½ cup heavy cream

2 tbsp. butter

salt and pepper to taste

Directions

1. Place spinach and onion to a pan with water and heat over medium-high fire.

2. Add stock cube and garlic and allow to steam for 8-10 minutes or until all the water has evaporated and the spinach is very soft.

3. Pour in the heavy cream and butter and then season with salt and pepper. Cooking until it thickens.

4. Using a hand-held blender blitz the spinach until fairly smooth.

5. Serve while hot

Nutritional Info (1/2 cup)

Calories: 200

Net Carbs: 3g

Fat: 23g

Protein: 7g

Chicken and Mushroom Stew

Ingredients

8 pcs. chicken thighs

4 tbsp. butter

3 cloves garlic, minced

6 cups mushrooms

1 cup chicken stock

½ tsp. dried thyme

½ tsp. dried oregano

½ tsp. dried basil

¼ cup heavy cream

½ cup parmesan cheese, grated

1 tbsp. whole-grain mustard

Directions

1. Preheat oven to 400F

2. Season chicken thighs with salt and pepper

3. Heat an oven-proof pan over medium fire and melt 2 tbsp. of butter.

4. Add the chicken, skin-side down, and fry both sides until golden brown, or about 2-3 minutes per side. Set aside.

5. Melt remaining 2 tbsp. butter. Add garlic, thyme, oregano and basil and mushrooms, and cook, stirring occasionally. Cook until browned, about 5-6 minutes, season with salt and pepper, to taste.

6. Stir in chicken stock, then chicken back to the pan.

7. Pour everything into a baking dish with the chicken.

8. Place into oven and roast until completely cooked through for about 25-30 minutes. Set aside chicken.

9. Transfer sauces back into the original pan.

10. Stir in heavy cream, parmesan cheese and mustard. Bring to a boil; reduce heat and simmer until slightly reduced, about 5 minutes.

11. Serve chicken immediately, topped with mushroom mixture.

Nutritional Info (1 serving)

Calories: 203

Net Carbs: 9g

Fat: 3g

Protein: 28g

Beef Shin Stew

Ingredients

2 lb. quality shin of beef

4 tbsp. olive oil

2 red onions, peeled and roughly chopped

3 pcs. carrots, peeled and roughly chopped

3 sticks celery, trimmed and roughly chopped

4 cloves garlic, unpeeled

a few sprigs of fresh rosemary

2 bay leaves

2 cups mushrooms

2 cups baby marrows

salt and pepper to taste

1 tbsp. psyllium husk

2 cans 400 g tomatoes

⅔ bottle red wine

Directions

1. Preheat your oven to 360F
2. In a heavy-bottomed oven-proof saucepan, heat olive oil and sauté the onions, carrots, celery, garlic, herbs, and mushrooms for 5 minutes until softened slightly.
3. Meanwhile, toss the pieces of beef in the psyllium husk, shaking off any excess.
4. Add the meat to the pan and stir everything together.
5. Add the tomatoes, wine and a pinch of salt and pepper and gently bring to the boil.
6. Turn off heat then cover the sauce pan with a double-thickness piece of tinfoil and a lid and place in oven to cook for 3 hours or

493

until the beef is meltingly tender and can be broken up with a spoon.

7. Taste and check the seasoning remove the rosemary sprigs and serve hot.

Nutritional Info (1 serving)

Calories: 315

Net Carbs: 7g

Fat: 7g

Protein: 20g

Bacon, Beef Sausage and Broccoli Casserole

Ingredients

500 g beef sausage

1/2 head of broccoli

8 slices of bacon

1/2 cup of cream

1 tbsp. Dijon mustard

100 g grated cheddar cheese

Directions

1. Preheat oven to 350F

2. Slice the sausage and place in a small baking dish.

3. Slice the bacon and add to the sausage.

4. Break the broccoli into florets and arrange between the meat.

5. Mix the cream and mustard in a bowl and pour it all over the casserole, then top with the cheese.

6. Bake in the oven for 35 minutes.

Nutritional Info (1 serving)

Calories: 300

Net Carbs: 3g

Fat: 25g

Protein: 20g

Creamy Haddock

Ingredients

150g smoked haddock

100ml boiling water

1 tbsp. butter

50ml cream

2 cups spinach

Directions

1. Heat a saucepan over medium fire.
2. Mix the boiling water with cream and butter in a bowl.
3. Place haddock and sauce in the pan and leave to boil until the water evaporates, leaving a creamy, butter sauce behind.
4. Serve haddock, covered with the sauce on fresh or wilted spinach.

Nutritional Info (1 serving)

Calories: 281

Net Carbs: 15g

Fat: 10g

Protein: 18g

Cauliflower Bake

Ingredients

4 slices of bacon

2 cups broccoli

2 cups cauliflower

2 cups mushrooms

1 green pepper

1 onion

200ml cream

120g cheese, grated

2 tbsp. olive oil

Directions

1. Preheat oven at 360F.

2. Steam or cook the cauliflower and broccoli until tender then transfer in an oven-proof dish.

3. Fry the bacon slices, with the mushrooms, green pepper and onion in 2 tbsp. olive oil.

4. Pour the fried bacon and mushrooms on top of cauliflower.

5. In a bowl, whisk 4 eggs with the cream and season to taste and pour over cauliflower or broccoli.

6. Place in the oven to cook for 25 minutes. Take out of the oven and sprinkle with grated cheese.

7. Place back in the oven and cook for another 5 minutes.

Nutritional Info (1 serving)

Calories: 100

Net Carbs: 7g

Fat: 6g

Protein: 4g

Caulicake

Ingredients

600 g cauliflower florets

1 onion, chopped

3 cloves of garlic, finely chopped

1 tsp. turmeric

100g parmesan cheese, finely grated

100g mature white cheddar cheese, coarsely grated

8 eggs

1-2 tsp. salt

2 tbsp. psyllium husk

1 cup of cream

1 tbsp. coconut oil

sesame seeds

olive oil

Directions

1. Preheat oven at 360F

2. Steam the cauliflower. Keep half of it whole and mash the rest.

3. Sauté the onion, garlic, turmeric in the coconut oil until soft. Set aside.

4. In a separate bowl, whisk the eggs. Add the cream, cheese, salt, and psyllium husk.

5. Combine the cauliflower, whole and mashed with the sautéed onions and egg mixture in a bowl.

6. Line a spring-form baking tin with greased baking paper and sprinkle with sesame seeds. Place the pan onto a baking tray.

7. Pour in the cauliflower mix and bake in the oven for 40 minutes.

8. As soon as it comes out of the oven, lightly prick the surface all over with a fork and drizzle with olive oil.

Nutritional Info (1 serving)

Calories: 160

Net Carbs: 5g

Fat: 11g

Protein: 8g

Burger Patties

Ingredients

500g ground beef

1 small onion, finely chopped

1 red pepper, chopped

¼ cup cheese, grated

1 carrot, grated

1 baby marrow, grated

1 tsp. ginger, grated

1 tsp. crushed garlic

2 eggs

2 tbsp. almond flour

1 tsp. parsley, minced

1 tsp. coriander

Salt and pepper to take

Directions

1. Mix all ingredients together in a bowl.

2. Form the mixture into balls and flatten into patties.

3. Roll the patties in almond flour and leave to firm in the fridge for around 30 minutes. This will help to keep the patties from falling apart while cooking.

4. When firm, pan fry the patties in coconut oil. Make sure your oil is hot before adding patties to the pan, you need to hear that oil sizzle. If the oil is not hot, the patty will stick to the pan and fall apart while cooking.

5. Take 1 large brown mushroom, rub with olive oil and some crushed garlic, do not salt. And bake in the oven at 360F for 15-20mins. Place the cooked burger on top of the mushroom, add grated cheese and melt in the oven for a couple of minutes.

6. Add 1 tbsp. mayo to finely diced red onion, lettuce and tomato and place on top of burger.

Nutritional Info (1 serving)

Calories: 340

Net Carbs: 3g

Fat: 28g

Protein: 17g

Slow Cooker Oxtail Stew

Ingredients

1.5kg of oxtail

1 Large pack grated cabbage

1 Large pack grated carrots

2 Large onions

1 Large Bunch of celery

1 Tin of tomatoes

2 Jelly Stock Cubes

2.5 litres of water

1Tblsp Crushed garlic

1 branch Rosemary

2 Bay Leaves

Directions

1. Place all ingredients into a slow cooker and cook on medium for 9 hours.
   Season with salt and pepper

2. Grate 60g cheddar cheese to finish (optional).

Serves 10

Chicken Hash

Ingredients

1 Tbsp. olive oil

1/4 onion finely diced

1 cups broccoli

1 cup chicken stock

50g chicken breast cooked and finely diced

½ tsp. salt

¼ tsp. black pepper

¼ cup pumpkin

Directions

1. Add all ingredients to chicken stock, cover and cook approximately 20 minutes

Tuna Fish Stew

Ingredients

1 tin tuna in water, drained

1 Tbsp. butter

¼ small onion, chopped finely

1 clove garlic, minced

1teaspoon fresh ginger, grated

½ tin tomatoes, chopped finely

1 cup spinach, chopped finely

1 small carrot, grated

1 teaspoon curry powder 1 teaspoon turmeric

½ teaspoon cayenne pepper (optional)

Salt & pepper to taste

Directions

1. Fry onion, garlic and ginger in butter.

2. Add tomatoes once onions are soft.

3. Add spices and enough water to make a stew for the spinach, carrot and tuna fish. Cook at low heat for about 15 minutes.

4. Do not overcook spinach.

5. Steam 2 cups of cauliflower, mash and add 1Tblsp of butter. Serve stew on top of the caulimash.

Ratatouille

Serves 4

Ingredients

2 large brinjals

1 large onion

2 peppers (can be green, red, yellow)

2 tins of chopped tomatoes

1 packet baby marrows

1 punnet mushrooms

1 packet spinach

500ml chicken stock

Salt & pepper

2 cloves garlic (finely chopped or pressed)

Directions

1. Finely chop all the ingredients.

2. Add all the finely chopped veggies, garlic and onion to the stock and boil on medium until the water has reduced, and the veggies have formed a thick delicious stew.

3. Serve with 150g chunky cottage cheese, 30g cheddar or 6Tblsp Parmesan Cheese

Easy Roast Tomato Sauce

Serves 10

Ingredients

10 tomatoes

Bunch of fresh basil

Garlic, bulb

Olive oil

Salt and pepper

Directions

1. Preheat oven to 190C,

2. Slice 10 tomatoes in half lengthways

3. Add a bunch of fresh basil.

4. Cut an entire bulb of garlic through the middle and place each half face up in the baking tray/dish

5. Immerse the tomatoes in olive oil and grind salt and pepper (Himalayan).

6. Roast in oven for about 1 hour and then turn the oven off for another 30 mins and leave to sit in the warm oven.

7. Remove the tomatoes and allow to cool,

8. Do not mix, as you want to squeeze the flesh and pips out of the skin and discard the skin, squeeze the garlic from the cloves and throw away the casings.

9. Mash with a fork

Note: This makes THE best roast tomato sauce for pizza's meatballs or any other protein. Freeze in small Ziploc bags or plastic containers.

You can add onion, red and yellow peppers and fresh chill for more robust flavour. Use a hand blender to blitz if you want a smoother sauce.

Tender Pork & Bacon Cassoulet

Ingredients

1 pack bacon, fried and then crumbled

Chopped onion (2 cups)

Dried thyme (1 teaspoon)

Dried rosemary (1/2 teaspoon)

3 garlic cloves, crushed

Salt (1/2 teaspoon)

Freshly ground black pepper (1/2 teaspoon)

2 cans diced tomatoes, drained

500g boneless pork loin roast, trimmed and cut into 2cm cubes

250g smoked sausage, cut into 1cm cubes

Finely shredded fresh Parmesan cheese (8 teaspoons)

Chopped fresh flat-leaf parsley (8 teaspoons)

Directions

1. Fry bacon onion, thyme, rosemary, and garlic, then add salt, pepper, and tomatoes; bring to a boil.

2. Remove from heat.

3. Place all ingredients in the slow cooker, alternating the meat with the tomato sauce until finished. Cover and cook on low for 5 hours. Sprinkle with Parmesan cheese and parsley when cooked

Servings: 4

Nutrition Facts (per serving)

Calories- 258

Carbs- 10.8g

Protein- 27g

Fats- 12.6g

Lamb Cutlets with Garlic Sauce

Serves 6

Ingredients

4 lbs. lamb cutlets

1 small head of garlic, cloves peeled

2 Tbsp. apple cider vinegar

1/2 cup water

1/4 cup extra virgin olive oil

Pinch salt and black ground pepper to taste

Directions

1. Crush the garlic cloves thoroughly in a mortar. In a bowl, add the vinegar and water and mix it well with the crushed garlic. Set aside.

2. In a large frying pan, pour the olive oil and fry the lamb cutlets until nicely brown.

3. Add the garlic mixture and let it cook gently for about 10 minutes.

4. Shake the frying pan to spread the garlic mixture evenly over the lamb.

5. Season with salt and black pepper to taste. Serve.

Cooking Times: 40 minutes

Amount Per Serving

Carbs 0,16g

Calories 416, 68

Fat 28,76g

Fiber 0,01g

Sugar 0,05g

Protein 36,68g

Tangy Shrimp Soup

Serves 8

Ingredients

12 oz. fresh shrimp, peeled and deveined

1 cup zucchini (medium, sliced)

1 onion, chopped

2 cloves garlic, minced

1 Tbsp. ginger, minced

1 pinch crushed red pepper

2 quarts water

1 cup celery (chopped)

2 cups cauliflower florets

2 Tbsp. soy sauce

1/4 tsp. ground black pepper

2 tsp. olive oil

Directions

1. In a large saucepan with over medium heat cook onion, garlic, ginger and crushed red pepper for 2 minutes.

2. Pour in water, cauliflower florets and celery and bring to a boil. Reduce heat, cover and simmer 5 minutes.

3. Stir in zucchini and shrimp, season with salt and pepper to taste; cover and cook 5 - 7 minutes.

4. Stir in soy sauce and pepper and serve.

Cooking Times

Total Time: 25 minutes

Amount Per Serving

Carbs 7,12g

Calories 107, 62

Fat 3,08g

Fiber 1,6g

Sugar 3,35g

Protein 12,08g

Baked Herb Salmon Fillets

Serves 6

Ingredients

2 lbs. salmon fillets

1/2 cup chopped fresh mushrooms

1/2 cup chopped green onions

4 oz. butter

4 Tbsp. coconut oil

1/2 cup tamari soy sauce

1 tsp. minced garlic

1/4 tsp. thyme

1/2 tsp. rosemary

1/4 tsp. tarragon

1/2 tsp. ground ginger

1/2 tsp. basil

1 tsp. oregano leaves

Directions

1. Preheat oven to 350 degrees F. Line a large baking pan with foil.

2. Cut salmon filet in pieces. Put the salmon into the ziploc bag with the tamari sauce, sesame oil and spices sauce mixture. Refrigerate the salmon and marinade it for 4 hours.

3. Put the salmon in a baking pan and bake fillets for 10-15 minutes.

4. Melt the butter. Add the chopped fresh mushrooms and green onion to it, and mix. Remove the salmon from the oven, and pour the butter mixture over the salmon fillets, making sure each fillet gets covered.

5. Bake for about 10 minutes more. Serve immediately.

Cooking Times
Inactive Time: 4 hours
Total Time: 35 minutes

Amount Per Serving
Carbs 2,77g
Calories 449
Fat 34,11g
Fiber 0,72g
Sugar 0,79g
Protein 33,19g

Slow Cooked Chicken Masala

Serves 2

Ingredients

1 ½ lb. boneless chicken thighs, sliced into small pieces

2 cloves of garlic

1 tsp. ginger, grated

1 tsp. onion powder

3 tbsp. masala

1 tsp. paprika

2 tsp. salt

½ cup coconut milk (divided into 2)

2 tbsp. tomato paste

½ cup diced tomatoes

2 tbsp. olive oil

½ cup heavy cream

1 tsp. stevia

fresh cilantro for garnish

Directions

1. Place the chicken firs in the slow cooker. Add the grated ginger, garlic, and the rest of the spices. Stir.

2. Add the tomato paste and diced tomatoes next and stir again.

3. Pour the ½ of the coconut milk and mix and then cook on high for 3 hours.

4. When done cooking, add the remaining coconut milk, heavy cream, stevia, and mix again.

5. Serve hot.

Nutritional Information

Calories 493

Net Carbs 5.8g

Fats 41.2g

Protein 26g

Baked Buttered Chicken

Serves 2

Ingredients

4 pcs. chicken thighs

¼ cup softened organic butter

1 tsp. rosemary, dried

1 tsp. basil, dried

½ tsp. salt

½ tsp. pepper

Directions

1. Set oven at 350F.
2. Whisk all the ingredients (except the chicken) in a bowl.
3. Place the chicken thighs on a baking sheet lined with foil and generously brush it with the butter mixture.
4. Place the chicken in the oven to bake for an hour.
5. Serve warm.

Nutritional Information

Calories 735

Net Carbs 0.8g

Fats 33.7g

Protein 101.8g

Slow-Cooke Stroganoff

Serves 4

Ingredients

1 lb. beef, cut into cubes

16 oz. cream of mushroom soup

1 onion, chopped

2 carrots, sliced

1 pc. bay leaf

1 tbsp. flour

2 tbsp. ghee

salt and pepper to taste

Directions

1. Season the beef with salt and pepper and then sprinkle with the flour.

2. In a cast iron skillet, heat the ghee on medium fire and then add the beef until cooked through.

3. Transfer the beef cubes in a slow cooker and then add the rest of the ingredients. Stir and then cover.

4. Cook on low for 6 hours. Serve warm.

Nutritional Information

Calories 345

Net Carbs 10.8g

Fats 16.8g

Protein 36.1g

Fiber 1.4g

Sunday's Best Roast Beef

Serves 4-5

Ingredients

1.5 lb. beef roast

8oz. cream of mushroom soup

½ tsp. chili powder

1 tsp. smoked paprika

salt and pepper to taste

Directions

1. Season the beef with chili powder, paprika, salt, and pepper.
2. Place the beef in a slow cooker and pour over the mushroom soup.
3. Cover and cook on low for 6 hours.

Nutritional Information

Calories 252

Net Carbs 6.4g

Fats 53.6g

Protein 15g

Fiber 1.2g

Sweet and Sour Snapper

Serves 2

Ingredients

4 fillets snapper

¼ cup fresh coriander, chopped

4 tbsp. juice of lime

6 pcs. lychees, sliced

2 tbsp. olive oil

salt and pepper to taste

Directions

1. Season the filets with salt and pepper.
2. Heat the olive oil on a pan over medium heat and cook for 4 minutes on each side.
3. Drizzle the lime juice on the fish, add the coriander, and the sliced lychees.
4. Reduce the heat to low and allow to cook for another 5 minutes.
5. Transfer into a serving plate and enjoy.

Nutritional Information

Calories 244

Net Carbs 0.1g

Fats 15.4g

Protein 27.9g

Squash Carbonara

Serves 3

Ingredients

1 pack konjac yam noodles (Shirataki)

2 egg yolks

3 tbsp. squash puree

1/3 cup parmesan cheese, grated

½ cup heavy cream

2 tbsp. organic butter

4 pcs. pancetta

½ tsp. dried sage

salt and pepper to taste

Directions

1. Boil water and soak the noodles in it for 3 minutes. Strain and set aside.

2. Sear the pancetta on a hot pan, and chop. Reserve the fat from the pancetta

3. Place the strained noodles on the pan cooked for the pancetta and cook for 5 minutes. Set aside.

4. On another pan (large sized) melt the butter on medium heat and allow to brown. Add the squash puree and season with sage.

5. Pour the heavy cream into the pan, add the fat from the pancetta and stir well.

6. Lastly, add the parmesan cheese into the sauce and the mix well. Reduce the heat to low and stir until the sauce thickens.

7. Transfer the noodles into the pan with the sauce, crack the eggs and combine all the ingredients together.

Nutritional Information

Calories 384

Net Carbs 2g

Fats 34.7g

Protein 14g

Fiber 2g

Macadamia Crusted Lamb Chops

Serves 2

Ingredients

6 pcs. lamb chops

¾ cup macadamia nuts, ground

2 tbsp. fresh rosemary

salt and pepper to taste

2 tbsp. ghee

Directions

1. Set oven at 350F

2. Season the lamb chops with salt and pepper. Drizzle with ghee on top.

3. Combine the macadamia nuts and rosemary and roll the lamb chops on the mixture.

4. Place the lamb chops on a baking sheet lined with oil and place in the oven to cook for 25 minutes.

5. Serve warm.

Nutritional Information

Calories 856

Net Carbs 9.1g

Fats 66.0g

Protein 60.3g

Fiber 5.7g

Chicken in Kung Pao Sauce

Serves 2

Ingredients

2 boneless chicken thighs, cut into smaller pieces

½ green pepper, chopped

2 pcs. spring onions, sliced thin

¼ cup peanuts, chopped

1 tsp. ginger, grated

½ tbsp. red chili flakes

salt and pepper to taste

For the sauce:

2 tsp. rice wine vinegar

1 tbsp. Atkins ketchup

2 tbsp. chili garlic paste

1 tbsp. low-sodium soy sauce

2 tsp. sesame oil

2 tsp. liquid stevia

½ tsp. maple syrup

Directions

1. Season the chicken with salt, pepper, and grated ginger.

2. Place a cast iron skillet over medium-high fire and add the chicken when the pan is hot. Cook for 10 minutes.

3. Whisk all the ingredients for the sauce in a bowl while waiting for the chicken to cook.

4. Add the green pepper, spring onions, and peanuts to the pan with the chicken, and cook for another 4-5 minutes

5. Add the sauce into the pan stir and allow to boil.

Nutritional Information

Calories 362

Net Carbs 3.2g

Fats 27.4g

Protein 22.3g

Fiber 1.3g

Asian Short Ribs

Serves 3

Ingredients

1 ½ lb. short ribs

For the rub:

1 tsp. ginger, grated

1 clove of garlic, minced

½ tsp. onion powder

½ tsp. red pepper flakes

¼ tsp. cardamom

½ tsp. sesame seed

1 tsp. salt

For the marinade:

¼ low-sodium soy sauce

2 tbsp. fish sauce

2 tbsp. rice vinegar

Directions

1. Whisk all the ingredients for the marinade and pour it over the ribs. Allow the ribs to marinate for an hour.

2. Mix all the ingredients for the rub roll the marinated ribs on it, making sure to evenly coat.

3. Heat the grill and cook for 4-5 minutes on each side.

Nutritional Information

Calories 417

Net Carbs 0.9g

Fats 31.8g

Protein 29.5

Chicken BBQ Pizza

Serves 4

Ingredients

1 cup roasted chicken, shredded

4 tbsp. BBQ sauce

½ cup cheddar cheese

1 tbsp. mayonnaise

4 tbsp. all-natural tomato sauce

For the pizza crust

6 tbsp. parmesan cheese, grated

6 organic eggs

3 tbsp. psyllium husk powder

2 tsp. Italian seasoning

salt and pepper to taste

Directions

1. Set oven at 425F.

2. Place all the ingredients for the crust in a food processor and pulse until you achieve thick dough.

3. Shape the pizza dough and place in the oven to cook for 10 minutes.

4. Top the cooked crust with the tomato sauce followed by the chicken, cheese, and a drizzle of the BBQ sauce and mayonnaise on top.

Nutritional Information

Calories 357

Net Carbs 2.9g

Fats 24.5g

Protein 24.5g

Fiber 6.3g

Margherita Pizza

Serves 2

Ingredients

For the crust

2 organic eggs

2 tbsp. parmesan cheese, grated

1 tbsp. psyllium husk powder

1 tsp. Italian seasoning

½ tsp. salt

2 tsp. ghee

For the toppings

5 basil leaves, roughly chopped

2 oz. mozzarella cheese, sliced

3 tbsp. all-natural tomato sauce

Directions

1. Place all the ingredients for the crust in a food processor and pulse until well combined.

2. Pour the mixture on a hot non-stick pan and tilt to spread the batter.

3. Cook until the edges are brown. Flip to the other side and cook for another 45 seconds. Remove from the heat.

4. Spread the tomato sauce on top of the crust, add the mozzarella and basil leaves on top and place in the broiler to melt the cheese for 2 minutes.

5. Serve.

Nutritional Information

Calories 459

Net Carbs 3.5g

Fats 35g

Protein 27g

Fiber 8.5g

The Perfect Baked Chicken Wings

Serves 2

Ingredients

2.5lbs. chicken wings

½ tsp. baking soda

1 tsp. baking powder

salt to taste

4 tbsp. butter, melted

Directions

1. Add all the ingredients (except butter) in a Ziploc bag and shake, making sure that the wings are coated with the mixture.

2. Place in the fridge overnight.

3. When you're ready to cook, set the oven at 450F.

4. Place the wings on a baking sheet and cook in the oven for 20 minutes.

5. Flip the wings and bake for another 15 minutes.

6. Melt the butter and drizzle over the wings.

Nutritional Information

Calories 500

Net Carbs 0g

Fats 38.8g

Protein 34g

Fiber 0g

Cauli Tater Tots

Serves 4

Ingredients

1 cauliflower head, cut into florets

2 oz. mozzarella cheese, shredded

¼ cup parmesan cheese, shredded

1 organic egg

½ tsp. garlic powder

½ tsp. onion powder

2 tsp. psyllium husk powder

salt and pepper to taste

1 cup ghee or lard for frying

Directions

1. Steam the cauli florets.

2. When done, place them in a food processor and process until you achieve a mash. Set aside.

3. Add the mozzarella, parmesan, egg, and the spices into the mixture. Also add the psyllium husk and then pulse to combine.

4. Using your hands, roll the mixture into small tater tots sizes.

5. Heat the ghee and then fry until golden brown.

6. Allow to cool for a bit before serving with salsa or sour cream as dip.

Nutritional Information

Calories 249

Net Carbs 4g

Fats 21g

Protein 10.3g

Fiber 4.5g

Malaysian Bone Broth Soup

Serves 5

Ingredients

2 lb. pork ribs, cut into cubes

1 whole garlic, crushed

1 cup dried shiitake mushrooms

1 cup enoki mushrooms

2 sachets. Bak Kuh Teh

pepper to taste

3L water

Directions

1. Bring the water into a boil with the Bak Kuh Teh sachets in it.

2. When boiling, place the ribs in the pot and reduce the heat.

3. Throw the crushed garlic into the pot and then add the mushrooms. Stir.

4. Cook for 1 hour or a few minutes more.

5. Serve hot.

Nutritional Information

Calories 517

Net Carbs 5.0g

Fats 32.2g

Protein 48.8g

Fiber 1.0g

Bacon Layered Lasagna

Serves 2

Ingredients

8 bacon strips

¼ cup all-natural pizza sauce

¼ lb. ground beef

1 cup mozzarella cheese, shredded

3 tbsp. parmesan cheese, grated

1 tsp. Italian seasoning

Directions

1. Set oven at 350F

2. In a pan, brown the beef over medium heat.

3. Drain the fat from the beef when cooked and then sprinkle with the Italian seasoning.

4. Layer 4 strips of bacon on a 9-inch baking dish and then spread half of the pizza sauce on top. Add the half of the ground beef and half of the mozzarella and parmesan and the cover with the remaining pcs. of bacon and repeat the process.

5. Place in the oven to bake for 12-15 minutes or until the cheese has melted.

Nutritional Information

Calories 702

Net Carbs 10g

Fats 41g

Protein 75g

Pulled Pork Shoulder

Serves 4-5

Ingredients

2 lbs. whole pork shoulder

2 tsp. paprika

1 tsp. salt

1 tsp. pepper

½ tsp. cumin

¼ tsp. cinnamon

Directions

1. Set the oven at 450F.

2. Score the skin of the pork with a sharp knife.

3. Combine all of the ingredients of the rub and then smother it over the pork.

4. Place in a baking dish and cook in the oven for 3o mins.

5. Take off from the oven and cover the dish with a foil.

6. Lower the heat to 350F and place the covered dish in the oven to cook for another 4 hours and 30 mins.

7. Take the pork out of the oven and pull using forks. Serve with a low-card BBQ sauce.

Nutritional Information

Calories 534

Net Carbs 0.9g

Fats 39.0g

Protein 42.4g

Fiber 0.5g

Loaded Meatloaf

Serves 4

Ingredients

200g prosciutto, sliced thin

200 g provolone, sliced thin

2 cups baby spinach

1 cup tomato sauce

½ cup tomato paste

1 tbsp. apple cider vinegar

4 tbsp. stevia

1 lb. ground pork

½ onion, chopped

½ cup bell pepper, chopped

2 cloves of garlic, minced

¼ cup parmesan cheese, grated

2 organic eggs

1 tsp. oregano, dried

1 tsp. basil, dried

salt and pepper to taste

1 tbsp. butter

Directions

1. Set the oven at 350F.

2. Melt the butter on a pan over medium fire. Throw in the baby spinach and season with salt and pepper. Cook until the leaves wilt.

3. In a bowl combine the tomato sauce and paste, along with the apple cider and stevia. Stir and set aside.

4. In another bowl, combine the pork, onion, bell pepper, garlic, parmesan, and herbs. Mix well.

5. Lay a parchment paper about 10 inches and spread the meat on top. Arrange the prosciutto on top followed by the spinach and provolone to create a meatloaf. Seal sides.

6. Place the meatloaf on a loaf pan lined with foil and pour the tomato sauce on top.

7. Bake in the oven for a little over an hour or until the inner temperature reaches. 165F.

Nutritional Information

Calories 516

Net Carbs 8g

Fats 37g

Protein 37g

Chicken Pie

Serves 5

Ingredients

½ lb. boneless chicken thighs,
cut into small pieces

100g bacon, chopped

1 pc. carrot, chopped

¼ cup parsley, chopped

1 cup heavy cream

2 pcs. onion leeks, chopped

1 cup white wine

1 tbsp. olive oil

salt and pepper to taste

For the crust

1 cup almond meal

2 tbsp. water

1 tbsp. stevia

1 ½ tbsp. butter

½ tsp. salt

Directions

1. Prepare the crust first by combining all its ingredients. Set aside.

2. Heat the olive oil on a pan over medium-high fire. Throw in the chopped leeks and stir. Transfer on a plate.

3. Throw in the chicken meat and bacon and cook until brown and add the leeks.

4. Add the carrots and pour the white wine and then reduce the heat to medium.

5. Add the parsley and pour the heavy cream in stir well. Transfer into a baking disk.

6. Cover with the prepared crust and place in the oven to cook until the crust turns golden brown and crispy.

7. Allow to rest for 20 minutes before serving.

Nutritional Information

Calories 396

Net Carbs 6.5g

Fats 33g

Protein 12.1g

Fiber 2.5g

Atkins-Friendly Pad Thai

Serves 4

Ingredients

3 pcs. boneless and skinless chicken thighs

2 packs konjac yam noodles (Shirataki)

2 organic eggs

¼ cup cilantro, chopped

½ cup mung bean sprouts

3 pcs. green onions, chopped

2 tbsp. peanuts, chopped

4 tbsp. melted coconut oil

For the sauce:

4 tbsp. lime juice

2 cloves of garlic, minced

1 tbsp. all-natural peanut butter

½ tsp. Worcestershire sauce

1 ½ low-sugar catsup

3 tbsp. fish sauce

1 ½ tbsp. sambal olek

1 tsp. rice wine vinegar

7 drops liquid stevia

Directions

1. Whisk all the ingredients of the sauce in the bowl. Set aside.

2. Drain the noodles in boiling water for 5 times and then dry using a clean towel cloth.

3. Heat the coconut oil on a pan over medium-high. When the pan is hot, sear the chicken on both sides. Set aside and allow the chicken to rest for a few minutes.

4. Using the same pan throw in the noodles and fry for 6-8 minutes. Crack the eggs on top and scramble with the noodles.

5. Add the sauce into the pan along with the cilantro, mung bean sprouts, and green onions and cook for another 7-10 mins.

6. Garnish with the chopped peanuts on top.

Nutritional Information

Calories 310

Net Carbs 3.8g

Fats 14.9g

Protein 39.3g

Fiber 0.7g

Classic Chicken Parmigiana

Serves 2

Ingredients

2 pcs boneless chicken thighs

8 strips of bacon, chopped

½ cup parmesan cheese, grated

½ cup mozzarella cheese, shredded

1 organic egg

1 200g canned diced tomato

Directions

1. Set the oven at 450F.

2. Tenderize the chicken and set aside.

3. Place the parmesan cheese on a plate.

4. Crack the egg in a bowl and whisk. And dip the chicken in it.

5. Transfer to the plate with cheese and coat the chicken with the parmesan.

6. Grease the baking sheet with butter, place the chicken thighs and bake in the oven for 30-40 minutes.

7. While waiting for the chicken to bake, cook the bacon.

8. Pour the tomatoes with the bacon and stir. Reduce the heat to low and allow to simmer and reduce.

9. Remove the chicken from the oven when done and ladle over the tomato sauce.

10. Sprinkle with the mozzarella on top and place back in the oven to melt the cheese.

11. Serve hot.

Nutritional Information

Calories 826

Net Carbs 6.2g

Fats 50.3g

Protein 83.2g

Fiber 1.2g

Turkey Leg Roast

Makes 4

Ingredients

2 pcs. turkey legs

2 tbsp. ghee

For the rub:

¼ tsp. cayenne

½ tsp. thyme, dried

½ tsp. ancho chili powder

½ tsp. garlic powder

½ tsp. onion powder

1 tsp. liquid smoke

1 tsp. Worcestershire

salt and pepper to taste

Directions

1. Set the oven at 350F.

2. Combine all the ingredients for the rub in a bowl. Whisk well.

3. Dry the turkey legs with a clean towel and generously rub it with the spice mixture.

4. Heat the ghee over medium-high fire in a cast iron skillet and then sear the turkey legs for 2 minutes on each side.

5. Place the turkey in oven to bake for one hour.

Nutritional Information

Calories 382

Net Carbs 0.8g

Fats 22.5g

Protein 44g

Fiber 0g

Cheeseburger Soup Indulgence

Serves 5

Ingredients

5 strips of bacon, cooked and crumbled

350g ground beef

3 cups beef broth

2 tbsp. organic butter

½ tsp. onion powder

½ tsp. garlic powder

2 tsp. Dijon mustard

1 ½ tsp. salt

½ tsp. pepper

½ tsp. red pepper flakes

1 tsp. cumin

1 tsp. chili powder

2 ½ tbsp. tomato paste

¼ cup pickles, diced

1 cup cheddar cheese, shredded

¼ cream cheese

½ cup heavy cream

Directions

1. Using the same pan where the bacon was cooked, add the ground beef and cooked until done.

2. Place the browned beef into a pot and add the butter and the spices. Cook for 45 seconds.

3. Pour in the beef broth, cheddar, tomato paste, diced pickles and cook until the cheese melts.

4. Cover the pot and cook for 30 mins. on low heat.

5. Turn off the heat and add the heavy cream and cream cheese on top and garnish with the bacon.

Nutritional Information

Calories 572

Net Carbs 3.4g

Fats 3.4g

Protein 23.4g

Fiber 0.8g

Sirloin Tip Cut with Cilantro Sauce

Serves 3

Ingredients

1 lb. Sirloin tip cut

For the marinade:

¼ cup low-sodium soy sauce

4 tbsp. lime juice

2 cloves of garlic minced

½ cup cilantro

¼ tsp. chili pepper flakes

¼ cup olive oil

For the sauce:

¼ cup olive oil

2 cloves of garlic, minced

1 cup fresh cilantro

2 tbsp. lemon juice

½ tsp. coriander

½ tsp. cumin

½ tsp. salt

Directions

1. Place all the ingredients for the marinade in a Ziploc bag. Add the beef, shake and then marinate in the fridge for at least 45 minutes.

2. Make the sauce while waiting for the beef to marinate. Add all the ingredients for the paste in a food processor and pulse until you achieve a smooth paste.

3. After marinating, sear the sirloin on a hot cast iron skillet heated over medium-high fire.

4. Cook for 3-4 minutes on each side.

Nutritional Information

Calories 174

Net Carbs 2.8g

Fats 18.7g

Protein 32.2g

Fiber 1.0g

Slow-Cooked Greek Chicken

Serves 4

Ingredients

4 pcs. boneless chicken thighs

3 cloves of garlic, minced

3 tbsp. lemon juice

1 ½ cups hot water

2 cubes chicken bouillon

3 tbsp. Greek rub

Directions

1. Coat the slow cooker with cooking spray
2. Season the chicken with the Greek rub followed by the minced garlic.
3. Transfer the chicken on the slow cooker and sprinkle with lemon juice on top.
4. Crumble the chicken cubes and put in the slow cooker. Pour the water and stir.
5. Cover and cook on low for 6-7 hours.

Nutritional Information

Calories 140

Net Carbs 2.2g

Fats 5.7g

Protein 18.6g

Roasted Bacon-Wrapped Chicken

Serves 5-6

Ingredients

1 whole dressed chicken

10 strips of bacon

3 sprigs fresh thyme

2 pcs lime

salt and pepper to taste

Directions

1. Set the oven at 500F.

2. Thoroughly rinse the chicken and stuff it with the lime and thyme sprigs.

3. Season the chicken with salt and pepper and then wrap the chicken with the bacon.

4. Season again with salt and pepper and then place on a roasting ray on top of a baking sheet (make sure to catch the juices) and place in the oven to roast for 15 minutes.

5. Lower the temperature to 350F and then roast for another 45 minutes.

6. Remove the chicken from the oven, cover with foil and set aside for 15 minutes.

7. Take the juices from the tray and place in a saucepan. Bring to a boil over high heat and use an immersion blending to mix all the "good stuff" from the juice.

8. Serve the chicken with the sauce on the side.

Nutritional Information

Calories 375

Net Carbs 2.4g

Fats 29.8g

Protein 24.5g

Fiber 0.9g

Make-Ahead Lamb

Serves 3

Ingredients

1 lb. leg of lam

2 tbsp. Dijon mustard

3 cloves of garlic

3 sprigs of thyme

½ tsp. rosemary, dried

3 pcs. mint leaves

1 tbsp. liquid stevia

¼ cup olive oil

salt and pepper to taste

Directions

1. Cut large slits on the leg of lamb and place in a slow cooker.

2. Combine the mustard, olive oil, and stevia and then rub over the lamb. Season with salt and pepper.

3. Inset the garlic and rosemary of the slits.

4. Cover and cook on low for 7 hours.

5. Add the mint leaves and thyme after 7 hours and cook for another hour.

Nutritional Information

Calories 413

Net Carbs 0.5g

Fats 35.2g

Protein 26g

Fiber 0g

Ground Chicken Satay

Serves 3

Ingredients

1 lb. ground chicken

4 tbsp. low-sodium soy sauce

3 tbsp. all-natural peanut butter

1 tbsp. lime juice

¼ tsp. cayenne pepper

¼ tsp. smoked paprika

1 tbsp. rice vinegar

1 tbsp. liquid stevia

2 tsp. chili paste

1 clove of garlic minced

2 tsp. sesame oil

2 green onions, chopped

1/3 bell pepper, chopped

Directions

1. Drizzle the sesame oil on a pan over medium-high fire.

2. Add the ground chicken and the rest of the ingredients and mix well. Cook until the chicken is done.

3. Serve with the green onions and bell pepper on top.

Nutritional Information

Calories 393

Net Carbs 3.7g

Fats 23g

Protein 35g

Fiber 7g

Spiced Beef

Serves 4

Ingredients

1 1/2 lbs. ground beef

½ cup red wine

2 cups mushrooms, sliced

1 bunch of broccoli, chopped into florets

2 cups baby spinach

3 tbsp. Atkins ketchup

2 tbsp. low-sodium soy sauce

2 cloves of garlic, chopped

1 tsp. cayenne

2 tsp. cumin

½ tsp. onion powder

2 tsp. ginger, minced

salt and pepper to taste

Directions

1. Heat a cast iron skillet and add the ground beef. Brown the beef before adding the minced ginger and chopped garlic. Stir well.
2. Add the broccoli to the pan as well as the spices and mix well.
3. Pour the wine, along with the spinach and mushrooms. Stir and cook until the spinach has wilted.
4. Add the Atkins ketchup, stir, and serve hot!

Nutritional Information

Calories 515
Net Carbs 6g
Fats 35g
Protein 33.25g
Fiber 12g

Crispy Curried Chicken

Serves 4

Ingredients

4 pcs. chicken thighs

¼ cup olive oil

1 tsp. curry powder

¼ tsp. ginger

½ tsp. cumin, ground

½ tsp. smoke paprika

½ tsp. garlic powder

¼ tsp. cayenne

¼ tsp. all spice

¼ chili powder

pinch of coriander, ground

pinch of cinnamon

pinch of cardamom

½ tsp. salt

Directions

1. Set the oven at 425F.
2. Combine all the spices together.
3. Line a baking sheet with foil and lay the chicken on it.
4. Drizzle the chicken with olive oil, and rub.
5. Sprinkle the spice mixture on top and then rub again, make sure to coat the chicken with the spices.
6. Place in the oven to bake for 50 minutes.
7. Allow to rest for 5 minutes before serving.

Nutritional Information

Calories 277

Net Carbs 0.6g

Fats 19.9g

Protein 42.3g

Fiber 3g

Pork and Shrimp Stuffed Peppers

Serves 3

Ingredients

1 lb. shrimps, peeled and deveined

1 lb. ground pork

5 pcs. bell peppers, chopped into quarters

4 pcs. green onions, chopped

2 cloves of garlic, minced

1 organic egg

1 tbsp. low-sodium soy sauce

1 tsp. rice vinegar

2 tsp. fish sauce

1 tsp. five spice

salt and pepper to taste

1 tbsp. sesame oil

Directions

1. Add the spices, onions, sesame oil, fish sauce, and egg in a large Ziploc back.

2. Throw in the pork and shrimps in the bag and shake.

3. Place in the fridge to marinate for at least 2 hours.

4. Set the oven to 375F when you're ready to cook

5. Scoop the pork and shrimp mixture onto the bell pepper, place on a baking sheet and cook in the oven for 35 minutes.

6. Turn the tray around and then bake for another 5 minutes.

7. Allow to rest for 5 minutes before serving.

Nutritional Information

Calories 91

Net Carbs 1.5g

Fats 4.7g

Protein 9.9g

Fiber 12g

Snack Recipes

Bacon & Onion Bites

Serves 12
Serving Size: 1 cookie

Ingredients

Almond flour (1 ½ cups)

Flax meal (1/3 cup)

Psyllium husk powder (1 tablespoon)

Onion powder (1 tablespoon)

1 large egg

4 slices bacon, cooked until crispy and crumbled

Sea salt (1/2 teaspoon)

Freshly ground pepper

Directions
1. Place all of the dry ingredients into a bowl (almond flour, flax meal, psyllium husk powder, onion powder, salt and pepper) and mix until well combined.
2. If you don't have onion powder, you can use dried onion flakes and blend them until powdered. Also, make sure you don't use whole psyllium husks - blend the psyllium husks until powdered if needed.
3. Add the egg and mix well using your hands.
4. Add the crumbled bacon to the dough. Process well using your hands. (Be sure to save the bacon fat from the cooking process for other uses - like some of the other fat bomb recipes in this book.)
5. Using your hand, create 12 equal balls and place them on a baking sheet lined with parchment paper.
6. Use a fork to press and flatten the dough.

Amount Per Serving
Calories: 109
Fat: 9

Parmesan Crisps

Serves 4

Serving Size: 5 crisps

Ingredients

Parmesan cheese (1 cup)

Coconut flour (4 tablespoons)

Rosemary, oregano or any herbs of choice, dried or fresh (1-2 teaspoons)

Directions

1. Preheat the oven to 350 Fahrenheit. In a small bowl, mix the coconut flour and grated parmesan cheese. Don't use finely grated or powdery parmesan cheese like you find in a canister at the supermarket, as it won't work well in this recipe. Try to find finely grated parmesan in the deli section of your supermarket, or even better, grate your own!

2. You can add any herbs you like. Oregano and rosemary work wonderfully.

3. Scoop a teaspoon of the cheese mixture onto a baking tray lined with parchment paper leaving a small gap between each. Place in the oven and cook for 10-15 minutes or until golden brown, but be careful not to burn.

4. Remove from the oven and let the crisps cool down before you remove them from the baking tray.

5. Enjoy!

Amount Per Serving

Calories: 233

Fat: 14.5

Mini Pizza Queens

Serves 6

Ingredients

14 slices Italian sausages

8 pitted black olives

3/4 cup Cream cheese

2 Tbs fresh basil, chopped

2 Tbs pesto

salt and pepper to taste

Directions

1. Dice pitted Kalamata olives and pepperoni into small pieces.
2. Mix together cream cheese, basil and pesto.
3. Add the olives and sausage slices into the cream cheese and mix again.
4. Form into balls and garnish with pepperoni, basil, and olive. Ready!!

Cooking Time: 10 minutes

Nutrition Facts (per serving)

Carbs: 3,5g

Protein: 10,4g

Fat: 23,43g

Calories: 261

Cheesy Bacon Balls

Serves 24

Ingredients

8 strips cooked crispy bacon, crumbled

1 cup cream cheese, softened

1/2 cup butter

4 tsp bacon fat

4 Tbsp coconut oil

1/4 cup Splenda to taste

Directions

1. In a microwave dish, combine all ingredients and melt slowly in the microwave until smooth. Set aside some crumbled bacon,

2. Pour into a dish or pan and place in the freezer until firm, about 30 minutes.

3. Before serving, remove from freezer, sprinkle with more crumbled bacon, slice and serve.

Nutrition Facts (per serving)

Carbs: 0,5g

Fiber: 0g

Protein: 0g

Fat: 15,9g

Calories: 151

Creamy Greek Balls

Serves 5

Ingredients

1 cup cream cheese, softened

1 cup butter, softened

2-3 Tbsp freshly chopped herbs (any combination of basil, thyme, oregano and/or parsley works great) or 2 teaspoons of dried herbs

4 pieces sun-dried tomatoes, drained

4 Kalamata olives, pitted and chopped

2 cloves garlic, crushed

freshly ground black pepper

1 tsp sea salt

5 Tbs parmesan cheese, finely grated

Directions

1. Mash the butter and cream cheese together with a fork and mix until well combined. Mix in the chopped sun-dried tomatoes and chopped Kalamata olives.

2. Add the freshly chopped herbs (or dried), crushed garlic and season with salt and pepper. Mix well and place in the fridge for 20-30 minutes to firm up.

3. Remove the cheese mixture from the fridge and start creating 5 balls. A spoon or an ice-cream scooper works well.

4. Place the grated parmesan cheese in a shallow dish. Roll each ball in the grated parmesan cheese and place on a plate. Eat immediately or store in the fridge in an airtight container for up to a week.

5. Enjoy!

Nutrition Facts (per serving)

Carbs: 2,8g

Fiber: 0,24g

Protein: 3,67g

Fat: 19,8g

Calories: 200

Smoked Turkey, Blue Cheese Eggs

Serves 6

Ingredients

6 eggs

2 green onions

6 oz. smoked turkey breast, chopped

1/2 cup blue cheese, crumbled

2 Tbsp. Blue cheese dressing

1/4 cup mayonnaise

2 Tbsp. hot mustard

1/2 rib celery

Directions
1. Hard boil the eggs, covered for 12 minutes.
2. In a meanwhile, chop up the smoked turkey breast and the celery.
3. Slice eggs in half lengthwise, scrape the yolks out into a bowl. Add the rest of the ingredients (except the green onions).
4. Grate the green onions over the mixture. Mix all ingredients together.
5. With the teaspoon fill every egg with the mixture.
6. Place on a serving plate and refrigerate for one hour. Ready! Serve and enjoy!

Cooking Times
Total Time: 20 minutes

Nutrition Facts (per serving)
Carbs: 3,9g
Fiber: 0,3g
Protein: 14g
Fat: 11,5g
Calories: 167

Pancetta & Eggs

Serves 4

Ingredients
4 large slices Pancetta
2 eggs, free-range
1 cup ghee, softened
2 Tbsp. mayonnaise
salt and freshly ground black pepper to taste
coconut oil for frying

Directions
1. In a greased non-stick frying pan, bake Pancetta from both sides 1-2 minutes. Remove from the fire and set aside.
2. In a meanwhile boil the eggs. To get the eggs hard-boiled, you need round 10 minutes. When done, wash the eggs with cold water well and peel off the shells.
3. In a deep bowl place ghee and add the quartered eggs. Mash with a fork well. Season it with salt and pepper to taste; add mayonnaise and mix. If you want you can pour in the Pancetta grease. Combine and mix well. Place the bowl in the fridge for one hour at least.
4. Remove the egg mixture from the fridge and make 4 equal balls.
5. Crumble the Pancetta into small pieces. Roll each ball in the Pancetta crumbles and place on a big platter.
6. Remove the Egg and Pancetta bombs in a fridge for 30 minutes more. Serve cold.

Nutrition Facts (per serving)
Carbs: 2,2g
Fiber: 0g
Protein: 7,5g
Fat: 22g
Calories: 238

Parmesan, Herb & Sun-dried Tomato Bombs

Serves 4

Ingredients
1 cup cream cheese
1 cup ghee
5 Tbsp. parmesan cheese
1/4 cup sun-dried tomatoes, chopped
1/4 cup Kalamata olives, pitted
3 cloves garlic, crushed
3 Tbsp. herbs mix (basil, parsley, thyme, oregano, parsnip, mint)
salt and freshly ground black pepper to taste

Directions
1. In a bowl, combine the cream cheese and ghee. Set aside for 30-45 minutes to soft.
2. After, mix the ghee and the cream cheese until well combined. Add the chopped Kalamata olives and sun-dried tomatoes.
3. Add in herbs and crushed garlic; season with salt and pepper to taste. Mix well with the fork and place bowl in the fridge for at least 1 hour.
4. Remove the cheese mixture from the fridge and create 4 balls. Roll each ball in the grated parmesan cheese and place on a plate.
5. Return it to the fridge for 30 minutes. Serve and enjoy.

Cooking Times
Total Time: 1 hour and 20 minutes

Nutrition Facts (per serving)
Carbs: 4g
Fiber: 0,5g
Protein: 4,6g
Fat: 14g
Calories: 157

Spicy Bacon & Avo Bites

Serves 6

Ingredients
½ large avocado
Butter, softened (1/4 cups)
2 cloves garlic, crushed
Crushed red pepper (1 teaspoon)
½ small white onion, diced
Fresh lime juice (1 tablespoon)
Freshly ground black pepper
Sea salt (¼ teaspoon)
large slices bacon
Bacon grease, reserved from cooking (2 tablespoons)

Directions
1. Preheat the oven to 375 Fahrenheit. Line a baking tray with parchment paper. Lay the bacon strips out flat on the parchment paper, leaving space so they don't overlap. Place the tray in the oven and cook for about 10-15 minutes until golden brown and crisp. The time will depend on the thickness of the bacon slices. When done, remove from the oven and set aside to cool down.
2. Halve, deseed and peel the avocado. Place the avocado, butter, crushed red pepper, crushed garlic and lime juice into a bowl and season with salt and pepper.
3. Mash using a potato masher or a fork until well combined. Add the diced onion and mix well.
4. Pour in the 2 tablespoons of reserved bacon grease and mix well. Cover with foil and place in the fridge for 20-30 minutes to firm up.
5. Chop the bacon into small pieces and place in a shallow dish.
6. Remove the guacamole mixture from the fridge and start creating 6 balls. You can use a spoon or an ice-cream scooper. Roll each ball in the bacon crumbles and place on a tray that will fit in the fridge.
7. Eat immediately or store in the fridge in an airtight container for up to 5 days.

Nutrition Facts (per serving)
Calories: 156
Fat: 15.2

Fried Tuna & Avo Balls

Serves 12

Ingredients
Mayonnaise (1/4 cup)
Parmesan cheese (1/4 cup)
Garlic powder (1/2 teaspoon)
Salt
Canned Tuna (10 oz., drained)
Avocado (1, cubed)
Almond flour (1/3 cup)
Onion powder (1/4 teaspoon)
Coconut oil (1/2 cup)

Directions
1. Combine all ingredients in a bowl except oil and avocado.
2. Add avocado and fold, use hands to form balls and dust with flour.
3. Heat oil in a pot and fry tuna bites until golden all over.
4. Serve.

Nutritional Information per bite
Calories 135
Net Carbs 0.8g
Fats 11.8g
Protein 6.2 g
Fiber 1.2g

Bacon Zucchini Fat Bomb Balls

Ingredients
1 lb. smoked bacon, crumbled
1 cup pork rinds, crushed
5 cups zucchini, minced
4 cloves garlic, minced
1 cup cream cheese
2 1/2 cup grated Parmesan cheese
4 oz. goat cheese
1 tsp. onion powder
1 tsp. garlic powder
salt and freshly ground black pepper to taste

Directions
1. Chop or blend zucchini.
2. In large mixing bowl, combine bacon, zucchini, cream cheese, goat cheese, 1 cup grated Parmesan, minced garlic, salt and pepper to taste. Mix until all ingredients are well incorporated. Refrigerate for 2- 3 hours.
3. In a meanwhile prepare breading; in a bowl, combine crushed pork rinds, remaining 1 cup Parmesan cheese, onion powder and garlic powder.
4. Remove the zucchini mixture from the fridge and prepare about 30 even balls.
5. Roll each ball in Parmesan breading mixture until well and evenly coated. In a frying pan heat the oil.
6. Fry the zucchini bolls until they are a nice even golden brown all over. Place on a serving plate and serve hot.

Servings: 30
Cooking Times
Total Time: 20 minutes

Nutrition Facts (per serving)
Carbs: 1,7g
Fiber: 0,25g
Protein: 7g
Fat: 13g
Calories: 151

Baked Creamy Shrimps with Artichoke Hearts

Ingredients
6 oz. shrimp, precooked
2 Tbsp. butter
1 can (11 oz.) artichoke hearts, chopped
6 scallions
1/2 cup mayonnaise
1/2 cup sour cream
1 cup Cheddar cheese, shredded
1 1/4 cup Parmesan cheese, shredded
1 Tbsp. garlic, minced
1 tsp. red pepper flakes
1 tsp. garlic powder

Directions
1. Preheat oven to 350F.
2. In a frying pan, sauté shrimps over medium heat with butter and red pepper flakes for 5-10 minutes. Chop the artichoke hearts.
3. In a bowl, combine all your ingredient and mix until well blended.
4. Pour the mixture in a baking dish and bake for 30 minutes in preheated oven. Serve hot.

Servings: 16
Cooking Times
Total Time: 40 minutes

Nutrition Facts (per serving)
Carbs: 6,32g
Fiber: 1,6g
Protein: 8g
Fat: 11g
Calories: 150

Blue Cheese Turkey Dressed Eggs

Ingredients
6 eggs
2 green onions
6 oz. smoked turkey breast, chopped
1/2 cup blue cheese, crumbled
2 Tbsp. Blue cheese dressing
1/4 cup mayonnaise
2 Tbsp. hot mustard
1/2 rib celery

Directions
1. Hard boil the eggs, covered for 12 minutes.
2. In a meanwhile, chop up the smoked turkey breast and the celery.
3. Slice eggs in half lengthwise, scrape the yolks out into a bowl. Add the rest of the ingredients (except the green onions).
4. Grate the green onions over the mixture. Mix all ingredients together.
5. With the teaspoon fill every egg with the mixture.
6. Place on a serving plate and refrigerate for one hour. Ready! Serve and enjoy!

Servings: 6

Cooking Times
Total Time: 20 minutes

Nutrition Facts (per serving)
Carbs: 3,9g
Fiber: 0,3g
Protein: 14g
Fat: 11,5g
Calories: 167

Olives and Sun-dried Tomatoes Fat Bombs

Ingredients
1 cup cream cheese
1 cup ghee
5 Tbsp. parmesan cheese
1/4 cup sun-dried tomatoes, chopped
1/4 cup Kalamata olives, pitted
3 cloves garlic, crushed
3 Tbsp. herbs mix (basil, parsley, thyme, oregano, parsnip, mint)
salt and freshly ground black pepper to taste

Directions
1. In a bowl, combine the cream cheese and ghee. Set aside for 30-45 minutes to soft.
2. After, mix the ghee and the cream cheese until well combined. Add the chopped Kalamata olives and sun-dried tomatoes.
3. Add in herbs and crushed garlic; season with salt and pepper to taste. Mix well with the fork and place bowl in the fridge for at least 1 hour.
4. Remove the cheese mixture from the fridge and create 4 balls. Roll each ball in the grated parmesan cheese and place on a plate.
5. Return it to the fridge for 30 minutes. Serve and enjoy.

Servings: 4

Cooking Times
Total Time: 1 hour and 20 minutes

Nutrition Facts (per serving)
Carbs: 4g
Fiber: 0,5g
Protein: 4,6g
Fat: 14g
Calories: 157

Pork Ham, Sausages and Cashews Truffles

Ingredients
8 slices smoked pork ham
8 oz. sausages
6 oz. cream cheese, softened
1 cup cashews, chopped
1 tsp. Dijon mustard

Directions
1. In a food processor blend chopped sausages and cashews.
2. In a separate bowl, beat the cream cheese and mustard until soft.
3. Roll the sausage mixture into 12 small balls. Take each ball and form layer of cream cheese with your fingers.
4. Refrigerate for about 45-60 minutes.
5. Roll each ball in the finely chopped smoked pork ham and place on a serving dish. Serve.

Servings: 12
Total Time: 15 minutes

Nutrition Facts (per serving)
Carbs: 1,5g
Protein: 7g
Fat: 11g
Calories: 125

Smoked Mackerel Fat Bombs

Ingredients
2 oz. smoked mackerel fish
2.7 oz. butter, grass-fed
3.5 oz. cream cheese
1 Tbsp. fresh lemon juice
pinch of salt

Directions
1. In a food processor put butter, cream cheese, smoked mackerel fish and fresh lemon juice. Blend until all ingredients incorporate well.
2. Line a tray with parchment paper and create 6 fat bombs. Place in the fridge for 2 hours or until firm. Serve.

Servings: 6
Cooking Time: 5 minutes

Nutrition Facts (per serving)
Carbs: 0,8g
Protein: 3,3g
Fat: 17g
Calories: 163

Bacon Fat Bomb Dip

Ingredients
6 slices bacon, cooked and crumbled
2 cups sour cream
1 cup cream cheese
1 1 cups Cheddar cheese, shredded
1 cup sliced scallions, white and green parts

Directions
1. Preheat oven to 400 F
2. In a deep bowl, combine all ingredients. Spoon mixture into a baking dish and bake until cheese is bubbling, about 25-30 minutes.
3. Once ready, let cool and serve hot.

Servings: 18
Cooking Time: 35 minutes

Nutrition Facts (per serving)
Carbs: 1,7g
Protein: 5,5g
Fat: 19g
Calories: 197

Turkey Bacon and Avocado Stuffed Eggs

Ingredients
6 eggs
1 avocado
6 slices smoked turkey bacon
2 Tbsp. mustard
1 Tbsp. garlic, minced
1 Tbsp. lime juice
1 Tbsp dried onion flakes
pinch Cayenne pepper, or to taste
1 tsp. garlic salt

Directions
1. Hard boil the eggs (about 12 minutes). Peel the eggs and slice in half lengthwise
2. In a large mixing bowl mash the avocado.
3. Scrape the yolks out into the mixing bowl. Add in the bacon, mustard, cayenne pepper, lime juice, onion flakes, garlic and garlic salt. Mix it well until smooth and creamy.
4. Fill every egg half with the avocado mixture. Refrigerate stuffed eggs for one hour. Serve.

Servings: 6

Cooking Times
Total Time: 30 minutes

Nutrition Facts (per serving)
Carbs: 4,4g
Fiber: 2,3g
Protein: 9g
Fat: 13g
Calories: 162
Protein 9,36g

Hot Pepperoni Bombs

Ingredients
1/2 cup Cream cheese
4 slices Pepperoni Sausages (or any salami made from cured pork and beef mixed together)
3 slices smoked bacon
1 medium Chili pepper
1/2 tsp dried basil
1/4 tsp onion powder
1/4 tsp garlic powder
salt and pepper to taste

Directions
1. In a frying pan brown 3 slices of bacon and Peperoni sausages until crisp.
2. Remove bacon and Pepperoni from the pan on a paper lined plate to cool. Keep the remaining grease for later use.
3. Dice Chilli pepper into small pieces.
4. Combine cream cheese, chilli pepper and spices. Add the bacon fat in and mix together until a solid mixture is formed. Season with salt and pepper to taste.
5. Crumble bacon and Pepperone slices and set on a plate. Roll cream cheese mixture into balls using your hand, then roll the ball into the bacon or Pepperone.

Servings: 6

Cooking Times
Total Time: 15 minutes

Nutrition Facts (per serving)
Carbs: 1,3g
Fiber: 0,11g
Protein: 4g
Fat: 16g
Calories: 165

Wrapped Bacon Rolls

Ingredients
4 bacon slice
6 toasted pecan halves, chopped
1/2 cup unsalted butter
1/2 cup of Mayonnaise
granulated garlic (to taste)

Directions
1. Divide bacon into 3 equal parts.
2. Spread generously each bacon part with unsalted butter. Press butter side into pecan pieces.
3. Top with each with a mayonnaise, sprinkle with granulated garlic and wrap in a rolls. Enjoy!!

Servings: 12

Cooking Time: 10 minutes

Nutrition Facts (per serving)
Carbs: 2,7g
Fiber: 0,15g
Protein: 1,78g
Fat: 17,7g
Calories: 174

Lettuce with Prosciutto and Butternut Squash

Ingredients
3 strips Prosciutto
1 cup butternut squash, cubed
1/4 cup sour cream
3 Tbsp thinly sliced fresh chives
6 lettuce leaves
Kosher salt and freshly ground black pepper

Directions
1. In a frying pan, cook the bacon about 3 minutes. Add the butternut squash and salt and pepper to taste. Cook, stirring 6 - 8 minutes. Add in the chives and adjust salt and pepper to taste. Let cool for several minutes.
2. Chop the bacon and add all other ingredients (except lettuce) and mix well.
3. Set the lettuce leaves on a large platter. Top each leave with a dollop of the bacon-sour cream-butternut squash mixture and then sprinkle with some chopped chives. Serve immediately.

Servings: 6
Cooking Time: 35 minutes

Nutrition Facts (per serving)
Carbs: 4g
Protein: 2,76g
Fat: 11g
Calories: 120

Pancetta Wrapped Provolone Sticks

Ingredients
4 slices Pancetta bacon
2 Frigo string Provolone cheese (or Mozzarela, Kasseri, Emmenthal...)
1/2 cup coconut oil for frying
toothpicks

Directions
1. Preheat your coconut oil in a deep fryer to 350 degrees.
2. Wrap your cut in half Provolone cheese sticks with the Pancetta. At the end of the wrapping, secure with a toothpick.
3. Drop the bacon wrapped cheese in the hot oil and cook about 2-3 minutes, depending on the thickness of your bacon.
4. Remove your Pancetta Wrapped Provolone Sticks to a paper towel to cool for a few minutes. Remove the toothpick and serve.

Servings: 10

Nutrition Facts (per serving)
Carbs: 0,42g
Fiber: 0g
Protein: 5,6g
Fat: 22g
Calories: 216

Savory Coco Bacon Bombs

Ingredients
8 strips cooked crispy bacon, crumbled
1 cup cream cheese, softened
1/2 cup butter
4 tsp bacon fat
4 Tbsp coconut oil
1/4 cup Splenda to taste

Directions
1. In a microwave dish, combine all ingredients and melt slowly in the microwave until smooth. Set aside some crumbled bacon,
2. Pour into a dish or pan and place in the freezer until firm, about 30 minutes.
3. Before serving, remove from freezer, sprinkle with more crumbled bacon, slice and serve.

Servings: 24

Nutrition Facts (per serving)
Carbs: 0,5g
Fiber: 0g
Protein: 0g
Fat: 15,9g
Calories: 151

Scrambled Eggs Muffins

Ingredients
3 strips of crumbled cooked bacon
6 six eggs
2 Tbsp Coconut oil or butter
1 Tbsp butter
1/4 cup softened cream cheese
1/4 cup shredded Gouda cheese
garlic & onion powder
black or white pepper

Directions
1. In small bowl, melt the butter and set aside. In a separate bowl beat the eggs. Add in spices.Heat some butter in a non stick skille on medium heat and scramble the eggs .
2. Put cooked eggs into another large bowl. Put in your cheeses and mix well. Add bacon and stir. Add the melted butter and coconut oil.
3. Pour the batter in mini muffin liners. Place on cookie sheet with or without wax paper, and freeze for about 30 minutes. Serve.

Servings: 8

Cooking Times
Total Time: 15 minutes

Nutrition Facts (per serving)
Carbs: 0,54g
Fiber: 0g
Protein: 7,9g
Fat: 16,9g
Calories: 186
Sugar 0,31g

Smoked Salmon Cream Cheese Balls

Ingredients
2 oz smoked salmon fillets
1/2 cup cream cheese
3 oz butter, grass-fed
1 Tbs fresh lemon juice
pinch salt

Directions
1. In a food processor put butter, cream cheese, smoked mackere and fresh lemon juice. Blend until all ingredients incorporate well.
2. Line a tray with parchment paper and create 6 Balls. Place in the fridge for 2 hours or until firm.
3. Serve.

Servings: 6
Cooking Time: 5 minutes

Nutrition Facts (per serving)
Carbs: 0,87g
Fiber: 0.1g
Protein: 3,29g
Fat: 16,62g
Calories: 163

Breading Kohlrabi & Bacon Rind

Ingredients
1 lb smoked bacon, crumbled
5 cups kohlrabi, minced
1 cup pork rinds, crushed
2 1/2 cup grated Parmesan cheese
4 oz mascarpone cheese
4 cloves garlic, minced
1 cup cream cheese
1 tsp onion powder
1 tsp garlic powder
salt ad freshly ground black pepper to taste

Directions
1. Chop or blend kohlrabi.
2. In large mixing bowl, combine kohlrabi, bacon, cream cheese, mascarpone cheese, 1 cup grated Parmesan, minced garlic, salt and pepper to taste. Mix until all ingredients are well incorporated. Refrigerate for 2- 3 hours.
3. For breading: In a bowl, combine crushed pork rinds, remaining 1 cup Parmesan cheese, onion powder and garlic powder.
4. Remove the kohlrabi mixture from the fridge and prepare about 30 even balls.
5. In a frying pan heat the oil. Roll each ball in Parmesan breading mixture until well and evenly coated. Fry the kohlrabi balls until they are a nice even golden brown all over. Place on a serving plate and serve hot.

Servings: 30
Cooking Times
Total Time: 20 minutes

Nutrition Facts (per serving)
Carbs: 2,5g
Fiber: 0,9g
Protein: 7,5g
Fat: 13g
Calories: 154

Common Mistakes On The Atkins Diet

One does not have to attend a class to know about the common mistakes on the Atkins Diet. Carbs as it is referred to in this context refers to food nutrient (carbohydrate) present in foods like potatoes, bread, pun cakes etc. The following are the common mistakes in the Atkins Diet. Getting the wrong information - Some individuals assume that eating low Carb diet simply means eating meat every day. This is wrong; everybody requires knowledge on how to reduce carbohydrates, the foods that have carbohydrates and eating a low carb diet.

Lack of sufficient fat

This could be mistaken for a low carb diet as a result of thinking that low carb means low fat. At the start, people can manage low fat dieting but as time goes this will

lead to them using up their own body fat hence getting hungry very fast. Therefore it is important to add fat to your body while on low carb diet.

Lack of enough vegetables in the diet

While on the Atkins Diet some people tend to forget including vegetables and fruits in their diet. This will be disastrous in the end because vegetables should be eaten in large quantities by one dieting on the Atkins and fruits that are low in sugar.

Eating Too Much

It is of no use to count the amount of calories on the Atkins Diet. This does not mean that one has to keep on eating and eating just because he or she is eating foods that are low in carb. You are advised to only eat when one is hungry and stop when satisfied.

Poor planning

Sticking in a new eating program sometimes might be a problem and one might find himself or herself doing what they used to do before. Therefore one is advised to plan before hand to facilitate free adoption of the new eating habit which means you will know what to eat and when to eat what.

Use of low carb packaged foods

When buying low carb foods that are packaged it is of great importance to understand the ingredients. Most of them contain maltitol which is bad sugar that is not required by a lot of bodies. Therefore this packaged low carb foods need to undergo careful experiments.

Lack of variety

Most people might find limited variety of foods that are low carb yet there are plenty, the only thing to avoid in low cab diet is sugar and starch. Every cuisine in the planet has a low carb variety; also most dishes can be decarbed.

Insufficient fibre in the diet

Eating of vegetables and fruits help in ensuring that one eats enough quantities of fibre. But forgetting or skipping to eat vegetables and fruits reduces the level of fibre intake in the body and this can be disastrous in the long run.

The Atkins Diet Lifestyle Changes

You are certainly feeling motivated to eat healthy Atkins foods to help you achieve your ideal body and to exercise more and you are now ready to make positive lifestyle changes that you are going to stick to from now henceforth.

You've probably tried to do this before but it didn't work out for you as you had hoped for. However, this time things are different. For one, you don't have to worry about getting ravenously hungry from a restricted diet. The Atkins Diet is the most indulgent diet on the planet and so making your goals this time will be easier.

However, it is important to note that lifestyle changes are a process that take a lot of time getting used to and you therefore require support.

The fact that you are now ready to make a change is a huge step; the difficult part usually comes in committing and following through with your goals.

Here are a few tips that can set you on the right path of success.

Make a plan that you can follow through

Look at your plan as a road map that is supposed to guide you on this amazing journey of change. Don't stress too much about it. In fact, look at it like an adventure that is going to impact positively on your life.

Be specific with every plan you make and most of all, be realistic. If your plan is to lose weight; how much weight do you want to lose and within what time period?

Small but sure

The best way to meet your goals is to start small by setting daily goals then let these transform into weekly goals. For example you can choose to replace your desserts with a healthy Atkins Diet food for starters.

Drop one bad habit at a time, don't go cold turkey!

We acquire bad habits over the course of time and so does replacing them with healthy habits this is the surest way to success. Take it one habit after another until finally you start leading a pure Atkins way of life.

Exercise reigns!

Earlier on we saw that exercise is one of the best metabolism boosters. You also want to tone up your body after losing all that weight and what better way than using exercise to get some beautiful muscles?

The important thing is to choose a workout that works best for you. If you are a no pain no gain' kind of person, then weight lifting might just be the thing for you. If you love adventure, hiking, outdoor running, rock climbing and other outdoor exercises will work perfectly for you. If you love dancing, you can join Zumba classes and so on. Make sure you get a workout that you will be looking forward to going to and not one that you will be looking for excuses not to go to.

Most importantly...

Your body is a temple that deserves to be well taken care of and nourished. Make your health your priority and you will always make the right choices for your body.

The Atkins Diet is the epitome of how you should feed your body. Don't be too hard on yourself either if you slip. Just pick yourself up and resume from where you left of. With time you will find that you will no longer crave junk and over-processed food.

Your body will be so in tune with the Atkins Diet you will only want to eat what you are sure is providing positive nutrition to your body.

In the Atkins Diet, we have nothing like cheating as all our foods are super tasty and super nutritious. The only thing you need to do is to commit to this diet to allow your taste buds to adjust so you can start craving healthy apple chips instead of the fat laden potato chips in food stores.

It's time to make the big Atkins Diet change!

Conclusion

Thank you again for purchasing The Atkins Diet: The Ultimate Guide!

I hope that this guide was able to show you that eating a healthy diet and leading a healthy lifestyle is as easy as eating fresh, natural and wholesome foods. This is all you need to finally lose all the weight that has been bugging you for the longest of time.

The next step is to 'spring clean' your kitchen and eliminate all processed foods and replace them with healthy Atkins foods that we have looked at in the book. Most importantly, commit to all the principles we have addressed in the book for the Atkins Diet to work for you.

Of all the basic tenets of our lives, health and food are perhaps the most important. Give the Atkins Diet an honest try and your life will change forever!

Finally, if you feel that you have received any value from this book, then I'd like to ask if you would be kind enough to leave a review on Amazon to share your positive experience with other readers. It'd be greatly appreciated!

Kevin Case